D1167543

A
DIRTY
WORD

A DIRTY WORD

HOW A SEX WRITER
RECLAIMED HER SEXUALITY

STEPH AUTERI

CLEiS
PRESS

Copyright © 2018 by Steph Auteri.

All rights reserved. Except for brief passages quoted in newspaper, magazine, radio, television, or online reviews, no part of this book may be reproduced in any form or by any means, electronic or mechanical, including photocopying or recording, or by information storage or retrieval system, without permission in writing from the publisher.

Published in the United States by Cleis Press, an imprint of Start Midnight, LLC, 101 Hudson Street, Thirty-Seventh Floor, Suite 3705, Jersey City, NJ 07302.

Printed in the United States
Cover design: Allyson Fields
Cover photograph: iStock
Text design: Frank Wiedemann

First Edition
10 9 8 7 6 5 4 3 2 1

Trade paper ISBN: 978-1-62778-276-0
E-book ISBN: 978-1-62778-277-7

Library of Congress Cataloging-in-Publication Data is available on file.

To my mom, who always said,
"Someday you'll be a published author,
and your first book will be dedicated to me."

AUTHOR'S NOTE

This is a work of creative nonfiction. The events are portrayed to the best of my memory. While all the stories in this book are true, some names and identifying details have been changed to protect the privacy of the people involved.

TABLE OF CONTENTS

1 | BEING BROKEN

The first time I used a sex toy, I approached the experience in much the same way I approached any terrifying challenge in my life: methodically, and with plenty of preparation. After brushing my teeth and retreating to my bedroom, I peeled off the layers of my day. I unzipped my calf-high boots and placed them in the closet. I pulled off my top, let my pencil skirt slide to the floor, and tossed them both into my laundry bag. I unclasped the diamond solitaire necklace my ex-boyfriend had given me—one of the few worthwhile artifacts of our ill-advised relationship—and placed it carefully in its box. I pulled on the articles of clothing I felt most comfortable in—my plaid boxer shorts and my soft-from-wear ARMY T-shirt. I locked my door.

At the time, I was living in a brownstone apartment in Boston, Massachusetts with three other girls. Outside my bedroom, it was chaos—the living room cluttered with a futon, a papasan chair, Christmas lights, a shiny black mannequin wearing nothing but a construction hat, and that Van Gogh poster every college student has, alongside one of Jimi Hendrix. Several tied-up garbage bags leaned against the wall outside my bedroom door, waiting to be taken out. Sometimes, when the other girls had friends over and they drank too much—double shots of vanilla-flavored vodka, a smell that still sets off my gag reflex—they would run down the length of the hallway and dive into the latest pile of bags with loud laughter, screams, and a final, crinkly crash. My bedroom, by contrast, was a sanctuary.

There was my small, twin bed pushed up against the exposed brick wall, neatly made. A dresser, pressed into a recessed corner. A drawing hanging on the wall opposite my bed, a piece of artwork done by a high school acquaintance. My books, piled up on my nightstand. When I wasn't out, I spent much of my time in there, reading in bed, sometimes with a box of pizza balanced on the windowsill. I had transferred to a college in Boston the year before with no friends, eager to get a fresh start after a difficult year back in New Jersey. Nine different people had cycled through the apartment over the course of two years, and I hadn't been close to any of them. Locked up in my bedroom, I almost didn't mind.

That evening, everyone else was out, and it was mercifully quiet outside my bedroom door. On my bedspread, lined up in a neat row, was everything I needed: a notebook and a pen, a bottle of water-based personal lubricant, and—most daunting of all—a large, purple, double-ended dildo.

The only other time I'd encountered such an object was at the end of *Requiem for a Dream* as part of a frenzied film sequence so disturbing you might forgive me for the negative associations it left me with. But while the star of that particular scene was molded into a single, extended line, this dildo was shaped like a lopsided *V*, its longer end about the length of my forearm.

I stood in the center of my bedroom, barefoot, my toes digging into the area rug. I looked at the dildo and swallowed hard, my throat dry. My temple throbbed, and my hands were clammy, and my stomach hurt the way it always hurt when I was nervous. Slowly, I approached the bed. It was time to get this over with.

When I grasped the toy in my hand, I found it to be both flexible and firm and, when I held it up, so shiny I could see my reflection in its lightly curved surface. But as I turned it this way and that, trying to figure out how best to proceed, I found myself with a bit of a conundrum: I had no idea which end was supposed to go inside me.

I looked at the instructions (because even dildos, apparently, come with instructions) and learned that the shorter side—with its bulbous end—was supposed to go inside me, where I would presumably hold it in place using only the strength of my pelvic floor muscles. Once my Kegels were clutching this shortened staff, I was then supposed to thrust the longest (and purplest) penis ever into a partner.

Oh.

Shit.

Um.

I didn't have a partner.

I schlumped back against my reading pillow, feeling defeated. I brought this dildo home from the office where I just started interning, and where I would be in charge of reviewing a variety of adult toys, films, and books. The plaid fabric of my pillow in its screamingly bright hues of cyan and cerulean and turquoise seemed all wrong in this horror scene that had suddenly become my life. The dildo flashed and gleamed menacingly. I sighed. What was I supposed to do?

After staring off into the distance for some time, the toy limp in my lap, my gaze shifted to my notebook. It still sat there, off to the side, an unforgiving reminder of that evening's purpose. I had a review to write. It was to be my first review ever. I couldn't allow a small technicality like not having a partner derail me. This review was my chance to prove myself.

I made a snap decision, grasping the shorter end of the toy in my hand. I would use it as a handle and slide the longer end inside of me.

That issue being resolved, I put the toy aside and turned to the lube next, unscrewing the cap and squirting a large dollop into the palm of my left hand. Earlier that day—after I'd announced my intention to review the dildo—the lead intern (whom I had just met) rolled his chair over to me, pulled open a drawer and, after a bit of searching, pulled out a tube. "I'd recommend using this water-based lubricant with that particular toy," he said, and I nodded, trying to act as if it were totally normal for a strange man to be telling me how to use an object that I would later be inserting into my vagina. "It's generally not advisable to use a silicone-based lubricant with a silicone toy," he said, straining to be as clinical as possible. "The material starts to break down."

"Okie dokie!" I said, nodding again as I took the tube and slid it into my purse alongside the dildo. My smile was manic. He smiled back, nodded in what felt like a gesture of solidarity, and rolled away. I was left to ponder the nature of my new internship, how I would eventually explain it to my parents, and what I had just agreed to engage in that evening.

Now, hours later, I cringed at how cool and slimy the lube felt, like ectoplasm or cold, congealed boogers. Eager to be rid of the slippery feel of it in my hand, I slapped the lube against the shaft of the dildo and stroked the length of it, wiping the excess off on my thigh. Then, I placed the dildo aside so I could crawl underneath the covers and pushed down my boxer shorts and panties, leaving them to dangle at my ankles. Finally, I gripped the short end of the dildo and brought the head of the shaft to the opening of my vagina. I breathed.

Its curved head was cold against my vulva and, despite the lube, rubbed up uncomfortably against my skin. *Easy does it,* I told myself, pressing it gently against my body. My body resisted.

Just a little bit more, I told myself, gripping it tighter and pressing with more force.

My vagina was like a fortress, unyielding, built to withstand armies, undercover operatives, and other penetrative devices. I closed my eyes tight. I pressed just a little bit more. I held my breath.

After a moment, I relaxed my grip, sick with the knowledge that I couldn't do it. That I couldn't let that imposing, purple penis inside of me. I couldn't write my review.

The next day, after confirming that no one else was home, I rinsed it off in the kitchen sink and then sterilized it in boiling water.

I never tried using it again.

Two years before, life had been different. I was studying journalism at a school in New Jersey, living in an apartment with three close friends and working a part-time job as a writer and copy editor at a local newspaper. And on top of that, I was in love.

My friends weren't crazy about Travis,[1] but they hadn't seen him at the beginning of our relationship—when he had been sweet and thoughtful—when he took care of me for an entire summer as I recuperated from a mystery virus that landed me in the hospital just one week after we started dating. He came to visit me there with roses and a shopping bag filled with paperbacks. He walked me up and down the hallways, just me, him, and my rolling IV pole. Though he was six years older than I was, I think he won over my entire family that week.

But two months later, our limbs tangled together on the couch in my basement, he said he wanted to have sex. I looked at him, struck dumb by how unprepared I was for this moment. Yes, I was nineteen, a late bloomer by some standards. But I wasn't ready.

Only a few months before, my mother had tried to have "the talk" with me, urging me to make an appointment with a gynecologist and get a prescription for birth

---

1 Not his real name. Most names throughout have been changed, for various reasons.

control pills. "He's six years older than you," she said. I sat on the living room sofa, running my fingers along the cushions and looking down at my knees. "He's going to want to have sex."

I glanced up. I could tell she assumed I would want to have sex right back. But sex hadn't even occurred to me. I was a virgin, and I planned on staying that way. I had been raised to believe in putting off sex until marriage. Why was this even an issue?

But there I was in the dark, terrified as he tugged down my shorts. The sound of his boxers whispering down his own legs was deafening. When he climbed on top of me, I held my breath. My thighs clenched together, and my vaginal walls tensed but, even so, he pushed his way inside me.

It was painless . . . physically, at least. Still, I cried when it was over and continued crying as I walked him up the basement stairs, holding the screen door open for him. "I hope you don't regret this," he said, choosing to ignore all evidence to the contrary. "I don't." With that, he turned away into the late summer night.

I watched him recede down the driveway to his car, into the night, the edges of him becoming more indistinct as the distance between us grew. My stomach roiled with shock and betrayal, and also the fear of what my mom would say. How disappointed she would be. It didn't occur to me that this wasn't my fault. After all, though I'd murmured the words, "I'm not sure . . ." at some point before he entered me, the words "no" or "stop" were never spoken aloud.

* * *

After that, it was like a seal had been broken. He had taken me. He had taken all of me. And because it felt like there was nothing left to preserve, I let him have me—again and again and again. "He's six years older than you," I remembered my mother saying. Which, to me, meant: *he needs this. He deserves this. And if he can't get it from you, there'll be no reason for him to stay.*

I wanted so badly for him to stay. I wanted to be his girlfriend, even after it became evident that there were a good number of things wrong with our relationship, things I had not previously noticed. There was his alcoholism. His jealousy. The way he could so easily manipulate me. But the things that echoed into my future, setting up permanent residence in my psyche, happened in the bedroom. The way he belittled my inexperience. The comments he made about my pubic hair, or my hushed quiet in bed. His obvious lack of concern about my comfort levels, even attempting anal sex with me *sans* lube . . . twice.

I remember one evening—before I became proficient at giving blow jobs, before I'd ever even given one at all—Travis kept pleading with me to go down on him. "C'mon," he said, not letting it go as I tried valiantly to enjoy the TV show we'd been watching together. I tried to ignore the queasiness in my stomach and the prickling of tears behind my eyes that came from feeling pressured, once more, to do something I wasn't ready to do.

When I finally made it clear I wasn't going to cave, he started sulking, giving me the cold shoulder. I eventually stalked out, sick of his impatience with me.

Eventually though, in the months that followed, I caved again and again.

Over the course of our relationship—a relationship that was only six months long, but which felt far longer—we broke up on four separate occasions. It didn't take, however, until my grandmother died. She had been sick for some time, battling lymphoma, in and out of the hospital, shrunken and insubstantial and nothing like the fiery woman she used to be. (Though she still had the wherewithal to mutter to my mother about how unfortunate it was that I was going to end up someday marrying this Travis fellow.) In the end, thanks to full-body radiation that affected her lungs and heart, it was congestive heart failure that killed her. I still remember standing in the parking lot of the funeral home where my grandmother's wake was being held, the late fall wind whipping my hair into my face and freezing my stockinged legs, on the phone with Travis, demanding to know where he was. "I don't do wakes," he said. "I don't really like them." As if everyone else in the world conga-lined their way to open caskets like they were on their way to Disneyland.

I had really needed him there. I wanted him to be there beside me, holding my hand, supporting me through my time of grief. And so, though I had allowed him to break me down again and again in the preceding months—taking my body for his own, leaving me unsure about myself and my abilities and my emotions—this is where I finally drew the line.

Considering his track record, I don't know why I expected any different.

* * *

Almost two years later—after I finally extricated myself from our relationship, abruptly dropped out of the College of New Jersey while in the midst of a panic attack, went to therapy for chronic depression and anxiety, languished in retail hell, applied and was accepted to another school in Boston, and then moved to a city four hours away—I interviewed for an editorial internship at an alternative weekly. The man who would eventually become my supervisor sat before me, riffling through my clips and pointing out weaknesses he perceived, leaving me wondering if I stood a chance. And then: "Do you feel comfortable working with adult content?"

What's adult content? I thought to myself.

"Of course!" I said out loud.

He proceeded to tell me about the two personals sites owned by the company—one of them pretty standard, the other more risqué and explained what his interns would be expected to do. He asked me if I was interested.

I realized this internship could give me back what Travis had taken from me. It could be a dare I gave myself, a sort of shock therapy. It could be a way to take control of my sexuality for the first time in my short, sexually active life, and put my experience with Travis behind me.

Of course, I said yes.

The first day of my internship, I was accompanied to the group intern cube and introduced to Mitchell, the stuttering young intern I would be working under, and

Amy, a sophomore at Boston College. "Here. Let me show you how things work around here," said Mitchell. He wheeled his way over to me and pulled open a drawer where bottles of massage oil in a variety of colors, scents, and sizes mingled with vibrating nipple clamps and sizzling body candy. My eyebrows shot up as I surveyed the plethora of pleasure products promising multiple orgasms and total bliss. Condoms—flavored, all-black, glow-in-the-dark—were strewn across the bottom of the drawer.

"Manufacturers send us their latest products, which we throw into this drawer," Mitchell explained. He closed it and opened the one below it, where I saw piles of eighties porn, Asian porn, and satirical porn, mixed in with erotic literature and self-help books on how to please your man. "We receive stuff from book publishers and film producers, too. Basically, we can choose whatever we want from these drawers, test it out, and then write a review." I nodded.

"That's pretty much it," he said. "Feel free to start placing dibs on stuff!" He wheeled back to his desk, bent over his keyboard, and started typing away at what I could only imagine was a salacious retelling of the latest post modern lesbian porn flick. I turned back to the two drawers and stared at them for a bit before finally digging in, pulling out plastic-wrapped items and the odd jar of something edible.

I sniffed massage oils, flavored lube, and aromatherapy sprays. I took a closer look at a couple of the books and slipped them into my purse. Then I looked at the toys still sitting there, toys the other interns were too embarrassed to take.

I didn't know the first thing about clit vibes, G-spot stimulation, or bondage, let alone what I might actually like in bed. But I was eager to impress the others with my progressive attitude, so I leaned deeper into the top of the naughty drawers and considered the clamps and dildos.

The Tantus Feeldoe, a shiny, silicone, double-ended dildo, caught my eye simply because it was purple. Purple had always been my favorite color. I once even had my childhood bedroom painted lilac (or, as the paint can called it, "demure"). I picked up the brightly packaged dildo, quite possibly the opposite of demure, and studied it. I then said, as nonchalantly as I could, "I've always wanted a vibrator, but maybe I'll try this instead."

When I wasn't at the office, or at the part-time retail job I also held to pay my bills, I was writing overwrought poetry and personal essays (thinly veiled as fiction) for a rotating array of creative writing workshops. My experience with Travis still so close I could feel its memory breathing heavy against the back of my neck, every piece I wrote was a fatalistic exploration of love and sex and coercion.

The poetry was especially terrible. In a poem about masturbation titled "Going to Town," I wrote that, after some fantastic foreplay, "you only used this as a sly vehicle / to get to your insistent thrusting that left me / staring at black spots on the ceiling."

I wrapped up the poem with a triumphant reference to my new love of sex toys and how I could "get me off better than you."

In one workshop, I read aloud a depressing poem in which I recreated the scene after Travis had taken my virginity: me, standing at my front door, crying, watching as his form diminished and eventually disappeared into the night. We had pulled our desks into a circle in the middle of the classroom, and I pressed the paper with my poem on it flat against the surface of my desk so no one could see my hands shaking. After I was done, there was a pause.

And then one of the other students leaned forward, raking a hand through her hair, and sighed. "I don't know," she said. "Your poems always make me worry about you. The fact that you regularly pair sex and crying seems problematic."

I wasn't sure what to say. It was a pattern I hadn't noticed. I pressed my lips together and made a *hmmm* sound as I nodded.

Later, I was taking the stairs down from the fourth floor with another girl from my poetry class. As we looped down, passing floor after floor, we came back to the topic of my poem. "You know," she said, "maybe Leah had a point." I looked at her expectantly, my hand sliding along the stairwell railing. "What that guy did to you . . ." She trailed off, thinking. "Maybe it wasn't rape," she finally concluded, "but it was certainly shitty."

It was the first time I had heard the word *rape* in association with what I had experienced. There was something about it that felt right, and justified, but a larger part of me dismissed it.

Either way, I didn't want to think about it. So I threw myself into my "work."

* * *

Failed Feeldoe experiment aside, I slowly warmed up to the idea of experimenting with toys and dirty films and of chronicling my own sexual experiences.

First, I puzzled over the Rabbit Vibrator, which had made it big after being popularized on an early episode of *Sex and the City*. The Rabbit was a phallic-shaped vibrator that pulsated and rotated and massaged my nether regions into a state of overwhelmed confusion. Though there was far too much going on there—especially considering that I was still hesitant about penetrating myself—I grew fond of the tiny rabbit ears sprouting out of the main shaft, which jumped and jittered, flicking my clitoris again and again. Clearly, clitoral stimulation is where it's at.

It wasn't until the Water Dancer, however, that I found true love. When it first arrived at the office, the Water Dancer didn't look like much. A waterproof version of the popular Pocket Rocket, it was a simple clit vibrator in a pale, translucent blue, with space enough for just a single AA battery. But then Mitchell slid that one battery in and twisted the base of the vibrator, turning it on. It jumped in his hand, taking all of us by surprise. It sounded like a lawnmower roaring across the vast expanse of mostly silent cubicles.

When I plucked the device from his hand and held it in my palm, I couldn't believe how strong its tiny motor was, how intense the vibration. "Dibs!" I shouted after we shooed away the office's sole IT guy, drawn to our group cubical by the sounds of buzzing and laughter. I took it home, where my orgasm blindsided me. Back when I was with Travis, he'd been the one to encourage me to explore my body. I masturbated for the first time in my life back then, amazed by the blossoming bursts of pleasure I could experience using just two fingers. But the Water Dancer was something else. When I touched myself with that tiny dynamo, a quick explosion of heat immediately flared up in my pelvis and rushed outward through all four limbs, leaving my entire body limp and tingling. After taking a breath, I brought myself to orgasm several more times in quick succession. Why would anyone not do this *all the damn time?*

But there was more to explore than toys. There was Crunch Gym's new cardio striptease class, where my supervisor sent me on assignment. Each week at class, we built upon a choreographed number set to the tune of Christina Aguilera's "Dirty." It started with a strut toward the front of the room, during which we pretended to smoothly pull off our tops. It progressed to a slap of the floor, after which we stuck out our butts and slowly ran our hands up our legs until we were standing upright. And somewhere in there we learned how to gracefully step out of our (pretend) panties. I felt ridiculous running my hands across my ass cheeks, looking provocatively over my shoulder to wink at my reflection in the mirror that covered an entire wall of the small exercise room. But I slowly succumbed to my instructor's insistence that it was okay to show pride in what I had and who I was.

And then there were the books that first exposed me to the intersections of feminism and sexuality. On that first day of my internship, as I dug through books in the naughty drawer with titles like *Tickle His Pickle* and *269 Amazing Sex Games*, I had been drawn to Carol

Queen's *Exhibitionism for the Shy*. It was written by a renowned feminist and sex educator as part of a movement I would soon come to know as sex-positive feminism. At the time, though, I picked it up simply because of the word *shy* in the title.

There were chapters in Queen's book on finding words that are hot for you and experimenting with dirty talk. Other chapters described how to maximize your pleasure, assuming you got off on being watched. There was even an appendix containing dirty words and phrases, synonyms for sex, masturbation, and various body parts (a goldmine, considering the work I was doing). But my favorite chapter was the one on awakening erotic personas. It appealed to me because it hinted at the power I had to change myself, and to change the way others saw me. Maybe I could see myself differently, too. Maybe I could *be* different. Maybe I could be the type of woman who had sex on her own terms, rather than giving it away, rather than letting it be taken.

In the bedroom, armed with a brand-new boyfriend, I began deconstructing sex as I was having it. Instead of submissively laying back and going with the flow when an intense humping session shifted into overdrive and the clothes came off, I now had products to test and new tactics to try.

"I never realized this part of the penis was so sensitive," I'd say matter-of-factly while simultaneously test driving the latest massage oil and full-body techniques laid out in Kenneth Ray Stubbs's *Erotic Massage*. "Do men really get turned on by in-and-out porn close-ups and bukkake?" I'd ask Darren while removing my panties, my voice carrying all the passion and allure of someone about to perform a prostate exam.

My approach may have seemed clinical, but seduction wasn't the point. Becoming an active participant in my own sex life, however, was. After all, I was trying to fix everything it felt that Travis had broken.

Darren didn't seem to mind. In the face of my open spirit of self-exploration, he became less self-conscious when up against the most awkward parts of sex, more open to experimenting, even when the experiments failed.

When I licked Pop Rocks-like sizzling body candy off his nipples and pronounced it delicious, he admitted that the feel of my tongue against his tiny nubs felt weird. When I queefed that one time as Darren attempted to get my legs behind my ears (an occurrence that is mortifying no matter how open-minded you are), he gave me this stricken look I couldn't help laughing at and said—soft and mournful— "Oh." Then we went back to it. Darren went with the flow. I was the one in the position of sexual power. It felt exhilarating. And while the relationship didn't last once I graduated and moved back home, it played a key role in those early days of exploration.

Other people treated me differently, too. One day, while at my part-time job selling kaleidoscopes and pug paraphernalia to tourists, my co-worker sidled up next to me. I was behind the counter, checking in new stock shipments and writing up price tags. She bent close, her voice lowered. "How's your internship going?" she asked. I had recently cut back on my hours at the shop so I could spend more of my days at the office on Brookline, brainstorming synonyms for "sex" and "penis."

"I'm enjoying it," I said. I shifted from foot to foot, glad for the momentary hush in the store, empty of customers for the first time all day. "I'm getting the chance to write in my own voice, which is nice." I smiled.

She smiled back at me, and then leaned in closer. Her waist-length gray hair swung toward me, creating a curtain between us. "You know," she said, her voice even lower despite the lack of foot traffic, "I write about sex, too."

I looked up at her, my raised eyebrows reflected in her reading glasses. My finger hovered over the price list in front of me. She nodded. "I'm a very popular writer of erotica," she said, "for an online magazine. I have a lot of fans." I looked at the calico kitten on the front of her oversized sweater. I looked back up at my reflection in her glasses. I opened my mouth and then closed it again. "Of course," she said, one edge of her mouth curled up in self-satisfaction, "I use a nom de plume."

"Right. Of course," I said, nodding, not knowing what else to say. At that point, the shop door opened with a whoosh, and I jumped. Two middle-aged women entered the store, shopping bags braceleted up and down their arms. We turned in unison to greet them before they walked off toward the back of the store where bird's-eye maple jewelry boxes mingled with laser-printed coasters. My co-worker leaned back in. "You're the only one here who knows," she whispered. She squeezed my upper arm conspiratorially. Then she left me there, alone with my price stickers and spreadsheets, to quietly consider not only her surprising side career in the sex industry, but also the way in which she'd marked me as a kindred spirit.

* * *

By the time I earned my BA, wrapped up my internship, and was packing up my Boston apartment before moving back to New Jersey, I had an entire trunk's worth of vibrators, erotic films, riding crops, and condoms. And though I had no plans to be a sex writer (my naively idealistic sights were set on such unattainable goals as "staff writer for *Jane* magazine"), I found I couldn't let go of any of it. Thanks to my new toys, multiple orgasms had become far more attainable. Thanks to my new books, I was learning a lot about feminism and women's sexuality. Thanks to the entire internship experience, I was feeling a lot less lost. Or at the very least, I felt as if I could someday find my way to a sort of sexual normalcy—to a place where I could enjoy sex rather than performing it out of a reluctant sense of obligation. It was an education I wanted to continue pursuing, even if only in my off hours, outside the boundaries of my career.

Two months after graduation, I landed a full-time job as the editor for an environmental engineering firm. I woke up early every morning, showered, and schlepped my way up the block to catch the 5:45 a.m. bus into New York City. Once arriving at the Port Authority, I descended two flights of stairs into the depths of the subway system, where I drifted along with the current of countless commuters down a long, gray hallway featuring Norman Colp's dismal "The Commuter's Lament / A Close Shave":

Overslept
So tired
If late

Get fired
Why bother?
Why the pain?
Just go home
Do it again.

This miserable piece of rhyme was laid out in pieces along the ceiling so that you came to the next line in the poem every few feet. Its tone matched my mood a little too closely most mornings.

After sleepwalking my way past this depressing reminder of my soulless existence, I climbed a set of steps to the southbound 2/3 line and boarded a subway train that traveled all the way down to Wall Street. After emerging from the tunnels, I made my way to an office building on Exchange Place, took an elevator up to the twenty-second floor, and then spent my days in a gray-walled cubicle, deleting redundancies in protracted environmental impact statements.

It was a far cry from the bawdy, playful atmosphere of my editorial internship. Perhaps that's why, after a time, I began using my emptier work hours to work on my own stuff. I sent my college-era masturbation poetry to a website that has, perhaps luckily for me, long since gone defunct. I wrote a piece about deciphering the line between sexy and sexual harassment in a work-place that produces adult content, and it was eventually published online. Even after being let go from that engineering firm and pushing my way into the book publishing industry, I still hungered to create more of my own work. I began seeking out continuing education classes, desperate for a creative outlet.

This is how I eventually made my way back to sex

writing, just a year or two after packing that part of myself into a storage trunk and leaving it at the foot of my bed.

While working on a class assignment that delved into the ideas put forth by Ariel Levy's *Female Chauvinist Pigs* (ideas revolving around women and the raunch culture that sexualized them), a woman I was interviewing invited me to one of her "sexy soirees." This was as far outside my comfort zone as I could possibly get.

But it was my experience at this party that led to a brief period of time during which I was active on the sex party/porn party circuit. It was this that led to my very first magazine clip: a travel piece on sex parties around the world that ran in *Playgirl*. It was this that led to my time at Nerve, my time as an editor at *YourTango*, my time as a sex columnist for both The Frisky and HowAboutWe. It was this that led to everything that came after.

And the impetus behind it all? The belief that this new experience, or that new experience, or the next one, or the one right after that, might fix me. The belief that the next crazy thing I tried would act as a sort of shock therapy to my undersexed system, making me want it more, want it enough, making me enjoy it—that whatever was broken inside me would eventually heal itself.

It was only slowly, over time, that I began to get an inkling that nothing would change, that I would always be this person.

It took even longer to realize I wasn't broken at all.

2 | BAD SEX

1.

I didn't want to date again after Travis. Though I had been the one to call mercy on the entire relationship, I could still feel the empty space of him in my body. The loss. The way I missed him. A gaping hole in the pit of my stomach. The way my heart hurt, sharp and wincing, as I occasionally wept so hard I choked on my own mix of tears and postnasal drip. Those tears left me wrung out, depleted.

I was reluctant as friends pushed me toward romantic encounters they thought would help me move past the whole, sorry mess. I wasn't yet ready to get close to anyone new, but I was intrigued and surprised by my power to still draw the interest of other men. It was as if they had no idea what a wreck I was on the inside. I carelessly blazed a trail through their hearts because it seemed as if I'd lost my own.

The first guy with whom I exchanged numbers after my breakup with Travis was an old friend of a friend. We met at a frat party in the basement, lights strobing, music deafening. I was trying valiantly to inject some energy into my dancing; to feel the way a person should feel when she is in the prime of her life and surrounded by free booze, catchy beats, and willing men. I saw him eyeing me as I performed my signature dance move: the side-to-side hip bump. By the heavy set of his eyelids, I assumed he was drunk. I was most of the way there, too, so I didn't mind when he edged up to me and placed his hands on my hips. He pulled me closer, his head inclined toward the curve of my neck, so we could exchange the usual pleasantries as we danced: name, school, major, etc. We shouted back and forth at throat-scraping volume as we labored to hear each other over the music. In the quick pulse of the strobe lights, I observed him in camera-click snatches.

He was my first kiss since Travis, and I didn't mind that it was enabled by beer and the sense of invisibility one can feel when hidden by darkness, erratic lighting, and all-encompassing sound.

But when we eventually saw each other again, things were awkward. He had just returned from a family trip to Mexico, and he presented me with a bracelet he brought back as a gift. When I saw that bracelet—a sign that this was someone who might be serious about me, someone who could care for me—something curdled inside me at the pit of my stomach.

I never called him again.

2.

Eventually, I fled to a different state.

First, I withdrew from all of my classes at my New Jersey college. This act was as surprising to me as it later was to my parents. I had always been a nice girl. A good student. Conscientious. Teacher's pet. But during the very first class of the winter semester—directly after the death of my grandmother and my breakup with Travis—I suddenly got the sense that I was in the wrong place. That I was suffocating. The professor was giving an overview of what becoming a hard news reporter entailed, oblivious to the fact that one of her students was scrabbling for breath, grasping the edges of her desk so that she didn't pass out. Nothing like this had ever happened to me before. Despite having been in therapy for over a year and being diagnosed with chronic depression and anxiety, I had never had a full-fledged panic attack. After rushing out of that class in a daze, I made my way directly to the bursar's office and dropped out of school. In this way, I thrust myself into in a state of limbo. I was still living in the apartment I shared with my three friends, who were all still in school. But I was doing nothing of consequence with my own life.

After dropping out of school, I did temp work. I worked retail. In my off hours, I lay in bed and cried, the shades drawn, the door closed. After a time, I decided I needed a clean slate. My roommate's mother had been making comments that my depressive behavior was adversely affecting her daughter—comments that infuriated me because *I* was the depressed one, dammit. I had also come to realize that a lack of a college degree wouldn't leave me with many very appealing career options. So I applied, and was accepted to, a college in Boston my therapist had recommended. I looked eagerly toward the start of my brand-new life.

When the time came, I moved four hours away from

home into a small room with one exposed brick wall in a three-bedroom apartment on a street lined with brownstones and hedge maples, just around the corner from Symphony Hall.

Just a month or two into my relocation, I went out with two of my roommates for dinner and scorpion bowls at a place around the corner. Their friend Steven joined us and somehow, he became the first guy I dated in Boston. The first guy I dated since Travis.

I'm not sure what it was. Perhaps the convenience of it all? He lived just down the block from us, and I often shuffled over there in my slippers to make out on his living room couch, to feel his hands move over me as we rolled around in his silly sheets, adorned with surfing cartoon monkeys. Sometimes I slept over and, when he kissed me in the morning before we'd even brushed our teeth, I'd think: *this must be love.*

It wasn't love. Though I was happy to let him kiss me, to let him rub his hands up my back, beneath my shirt, I continued to rebuff any of his more extreme attempts at physical intimacy. I wasn't ready. And maybe I sensed he wasn't the right match, the right man to take this risk with, the man who would treat my body and my sexuality with the gravity it deserved. Sex was a thing that was tied too closely in my mind to heartache and cruelty and manipulation. Did I trust him enough to wade back into all that? Was he the one who could change what it meant to me?

I wasn't sure, and I hemmed and I hawed and, perhaps because of this, I lost him.

One day, he never called me again.

3.

After Steven, I pledged a sorority. I felt isolated. I needed a quick connection. With someone safe. With someone who wouldn't want to negotiate me out of my jeans, out of my underpants, out of that place of detachment where I felt most secure.

I threw myself into the rituals of forced intimacy that exist among co-eds debasing themselves to gain entry into a closed group of females. Despite being a socially anxious introvert who typically avoided large groups, I made it to initiation night where I finally passed into active status. This evening culminated with an extended period of party-hopping, during which I kicked things off by guzzling Jägermeister from a large punch bowl planted in the center of a small, sticky, circular kitchen table. Leaving the third or fourth party, a fellow sister from my pledge class and I decided to accompany two guys back to their apartment located way out at the end of the orange line. I can't remember why we went, but they had probably promised me Kahlúa, or Malibu Rum. They were college graduates, one of whom also happened to be the older brother of a guy I lived with. We marveled at the coincidence as he stepped aside to let me slip into the back seat of a cab before him.

At their apartment, my friend retreated to the bathroom, and one of the two guys followed after, leaving me alone with my housemate's older brother. I sat on his living room couch as he brought out more drinks and, somehow, our conversation meandered its way to my sex life: to the fact that I had only ever slept with one person, to the fact that he had obliterated my heart, my body.

"I really respect that," he said as I sat hunched over, my elbows resting on my thighs, my head foggy with alcohol. I explained that I was waiting for the Right Person. I told him that I wouldn't let it happen to me again. That I wouldn't give away that part of myself until I felt I was ready, until I felt it was right.

He sat on the arm of the couch, perched above me, paternal, supportive. He said all the right things.

The apartment smelled of cigarette smoke and musty fabric, couch and carpet in disrepair. The back of my throat was sweet with the vast assortment of liquors, wine, and beer I had ingested throughout the evening. I can't remember how we ended up in his bed, grappling with each other, jeans pushed down to ankles, sheets shoved to the foot of the bed. But in that moment, I wanted it. I wanted to take this for myself.

But he couldn't get completely hard. He kept trying to press into me, but his penis was like a partially deflated stress ball and, somehow, we fell asleep that way: half undressed, sheets in shambles.

When I woke up just several hours later, dawn creeping through his bedroom window, I realized I was lying in a wet spot on the bed. I thought of Travis. Travis who had an alcohol problem. Travis who repeatedly got so inebriated he would wake up in the middle of the night and piss onto the carpet beside the bed.

I thought of Travis, even though I didn't know if I was lying in semen or piss.

I also didn't know if last night even counted. Was this virtual stranger my number two? Had I done it again? Had I let myself lose something to someone who—once again—didn't matter? Who would never love me?

I crept out. My tongue was a desiccated lump in my mouth. My friend and I rode the subway back into Boston, and I curled into the hard plastic of my seat, my hand wrapped around the pole next to me. As the early morning passed by outside, I felt fuzzy and throbbing and regretful.

4.

It seemed safest after that to close myself off. To flirt and fondle and kiss, sure. But to shut things down before they could get any further—which was tougher to pull off than you might think.

There was, for instance, the guy with the bad teeth who followed me home from Avalon, a dance club on Landsdowne Street. I don't know why I let him follow me into my cab, southeast to Symphony Road, through my front door, up the stairs, into my apartment, into my tiny bedroom.

I didn't want him there.

So I grabbed my toothbrush and toothpaste and left him sitting there on the edge of my bed. I took so long in the bathroom, spent so much time searching my face in the bathroom mirror that, by the time I got back, he was asleep on top of my bedspread.

I took a pillow and lay myself down on the floor. I couldn't stand to be near him, couldn't stand to let him think I was giving him permission, that anything was inevitable. When he woke up in the middle of the night and crawled down there next to me, I pretended I was asleep so all he could do was curl up against my back and drift back into slumber.

5.

There was the guy I met at yet another dance club while on a trip back home over Thanksgiving break. We spoke on the phone every night after that and one weekend he drove up to see me. When I wouldn't let him sleep with me, when I wouldn't let him take the one thing he assumed he had come for, he spent the next night with a friend before driving back down to New Jersey.

6.

I met Connor in my American Literature class. We huddled together at the back of the classroom, cracking jokes and bemoaning the tediousness of *The Golden Bowl*. We spent hours together in the college library gathering material for our research papers. We studied together at my apartment, seated cross-legged on my tiny twin bed, notebooks and textbooks sprawled around me like a blockade because I could feel him wanting me more than I wanted him.

I *wanted* to want him. I *wanted* to want someone who so obviously meant well and respected my boundaries.

But on the day he took my hand outside our classroom to walk me down to my poetry workshop (I could see my friend Matt arch an eyebrow at me from over his shoulder), I knew I couldn't spend time with him anymore.

He kissed me that day as he left me outside my workshop: a quick pressing-together of our lips. But I felt nothing.

Later on, after noticing that I was pulling away, he asked me what he had done wrong, how he could fix it. He apologized for pushing too hard, too fast, though all he had done was take my hand. All he had done was give me one kiss. I didn't know what to tell him. I didn't know how to tell him he had nothing to apologize for. I didn't know how to tell him that whatever was wrong was in me.

7.

Summer in Boston was quiet. Most students moved back home at the end of the spring semester so that they didn't have to pay the exorbitant rents and, as a result, I was surrounded by subletters: young musicians in their late teens who were in town for Berklee's summer music program. Two of them sublet a room in my apartment, and they had their friends over all the time to smoke pot and to talk shit and to record themselves banging on buckets and saucepans. Nearly twenty-two, I felt old and sluggish in comparison. I sequestered myself in my bedroom most days and, when I was feeling especially lonely, I went to a friend's apartment so we could watch movies together in his darkened living room.

Philip came along when I least expected it. My friend brought him over one day—on one of those rare occasions when my subletters were out—along with a DVD box set of all the *Godfather* movies. He was in town for the summer, working at the Gap on Newbury Street, and staying in the loft bed in our mutual friend's second bedroom. By the end of our *Godfather* marathon, there was an ease between us that was rare for me when it came to my interactions with new people. When the two of them left my apartment later that evening, I already wondered when I would see him again.

Looking back on that summer is like watching one

of those movie montages depicting a new and gloriously happy relationship you know will inevitably end. There we are, smoking on the rooftop of my apartment building, bare feet propped up on the roof's edge, the expanse of the city's other apartment buildings spread out before us. There we are, sipping smoothies on his work break, his collared shirt open at the throat to reveal his Adam's apple only intensifying the punch of want in my gut. There we are, dancing to the Breeders in the basement bar at Middle East, walking home afterward with our hands clasped together, acting unbearably cozy. There we are in the evening, perched on bar stools downtown, leaning in towards one another as I nervously fiddle with the straw in my whiskey sour. Where before my summer had been empty—all long, vacant hours of isolation in bed with books and magazines—now there was him.

I remember the first time he came over alone. Before, we had always spent time together in large groups of people, still spinning out that delicious tension of will-we-won't-we-does-he-even-like-me. By that night, my skin felt hot, hair-trigger-sensitive, the hairs on my arms reaching out to close the gap between us as we sat side by side on my bed. When he finally kissed me, it was like I had been holding my breath for days and could finally let it out, gasp in new air, breathe again.

But then Philip pulled the condom out of the back pocket of his jeans. The wrapper flashed in the soft light that shone through the window beside my bed. His bare torso, pale and luminous, slender, was striped with moonlight and shadow.

"How presumptuous of you," I said as I looked up

at him, my skirt hiked up to my upper thighs. This presumption almost ruined it for me. Almost put an end to everything.

"He tossed it to me as a joke as I was leaving the apartment," he insisted, referring to our mutual friend. "I swear, I didn't expect to use it. We don't have to . . ."

But I felt something for Philip that I hadn't felt since Travis.

And so, I let him.

Throughout the summer, I let him. Over and over, I let him.

It wasn't something I necessarily enjoyed. It wasn't something I wanted so much as I wanted his fingers entwined with mine, his arm slung across my torso at night, his knee pressed intimately, familiarly against mine as we stretched our legs out in the sun on the rooftop. The sex was never special for me.

But he was special. And so, I let him. Because I felt it was expected of me. Because I felt that he deserved it. And because I felt that he wouldn't understand if I said no.

Looking back, I suspect the only reason I let my guard down with him so fully is because I knew it couldn't last. He was moving back home to Tennessee at the end of the summer, and I carried no illusions that we would be able to sustain a long-distance relationship at that point in our lives. So, in a way, it was safe. I didn't have to invest every part of me into a relationship with him. I didn't have to worry that he would eventually notice my troubled relationship to sex. I didn't have to explain to him why I was the way I was, didn't have to watch him realize I was damaged, that I was too much work. Even at the end, in those last few weeks of August, I could feel myself pulling away. There was no sense in getting attached. If I cared too much, it would only hurt more.

8.

It was a long time before I felt anything like that again. There was a long line of men I held at arm's length as I squeezed my thighs together. Men who felt confused. Men who felt I led them on. Men who thought I was sending them mixed signals.

I didn't mean anything by it. I just wanted to be sure. And it felt easier to embrace my reputation as a tease, as someone who couldn't commit to one guy, than as someone who was afraid of sex or, worse, disinterested in it.

Four years after Travis, I was still haunted by his smirk, his scorn, the way he colored every intimate interaction I had. Though I had regained some aspect of control, for all my searching I had not yet found the key that would unlock the box of all the things I felt were missing. Desire. Pleasure. The sense of unselfconsciousness I longed for every time a man touched the small of my back or breathed hot into my ear or brought his mouth to my breasts.

So when I met the man who would eventually become my husband, I was still straddling a complicated line between Sex Writer Who Knows Things (an early iteration of today's Cool Girl, perhaps?) and Woman Who Has Lost Her Sexual Self.

When we first met, I was doing nightlife reviews for Shecky's, a publisher of city guides. It was an act of desperation instigated by my unemployment at the time. I was losing more money on bus fare into the city than I was making on the reviews, but the gig made for some fun dates. Our first week of knowing each other, we went out every night. I took him into NYC with me to eat duck at a Moroccan restaurant downtown, to prowl the floors of the China Club, chocolate martini precariously in hand. As much as I was floundering my way through my own life at that time, Michael told his friends that I made his life exciting.

Yet as much as we enjoyed each other's company, I still kept a safe distance. I made it clear to him that he was not the only name on my dance card. I refused to submit to labels like "girlfriend" or "monogamous." I told him that I was not the kind of girl he wanted to end up with.

The night he first kissed me, we were on the main floor of the China Club, backs pressed into a couch just off the dance floor, bare thighs sticking to the leather. I was nursing a cheap Chardonnay when he leaned over and pressed his lips to mine, his tongue slipping through the space between my teeth. When we pulled apart, I matter-of-factly announced that I was not one for public displays of affection. He visibly wilted, thinking I was outright rejecting him.

But later that night, we ended up in bed together. Pieces of clothing were peeled off one at a time until I was wearing only my black cotton briefs and, as we rocked together, he gasped into my ear, "If we don't watch it, we're going to get ourselves in trouble."

I felt myself pulling back in that moment, pausing. "I wouldn't worry about it," I said dispassionately. "I'm not going to have sex with you."

And in that moment, it made sense. We had only

known each other for a week. Refusing sex at that time was well within the parameters of "taking it slow." It was only when it became clear that this thing between us had some weight to it, some solidity, that things became more difficult to navigate.

I eventually slept with him. Of course I did. I was attracted to him and I wanted to, even if the intercourse itself never brought me much pleasure. But over time, it became more difficult to keep up with his desire for me. Over time, I could feel myself shrinking away. And when we found ourselves in bed one day, as he straddled me with a smirk on his face, I hesitated.

"Come on," he said, and suddenly it was Travis hovering above me, Travis squeezing his way between my straining thighs. It was then that I revealed myself to him, let the gleaming exoskeleton I had carefully constructed over the past four years fall away. I rolled away from him, tears rolling fat and hot down my cheeks, and he didn't know what was wrong.

I wasn't sure what to tell him at first. I had never known what to tell any of them. But because I felt that Michael wasn't someone who would drop soundlessly out of my life like the others, I decided to tell him the truth.

Darren, my easygoing boyfriend from my internship days, had never known what drove my bottomless appetite for sexual how-to books, my endless curiosity experimenting with sizzling body candy and sensual massages and wearable vibrators. He'd thought my clinical approach to porn-watching was all part of the job for me. Nothing more. And this made our relationship more fun for him.

But once Michael knew the truth, I couldn't play that part anymore. Not with him. And so, things got worse at first instead of better. Once Michael knew my truth, I found myself resenting him for wanting to sleep with me despite knowing about my past. Sex became so fraught that I started to experience a sharp, shooting pain during intercourse. A pain I struggled for years to fix though, over time, it became clear that it was most likely psychosomatic.

But still I slept with him, even though it physically hurt. Because I felt I owed it to him. Because I felt he deserved it. Because I knew I couldn't live without him.

Because this was love.

3 | OPENING UP

"Please don't break up with me!" he begged, his fingers tearing furrows through his hair, his usually pale skin deepening toward red.

I stared down at my fingers, my hands gripping the steering wheel as if I were afraid I might cartwheel away. We were seated in my car, parked outside the Barnes & Noble on Route 46, alongside a Dunkin' Donuts, a Kohl's, and a Dress Barn. We'd just had coffee at the in-store Starbucks, but our conversation had shifted in a direction that didn't seem appropriate for a public place. Now, locked up in this small, enclosed space together, I tried to push aside the memory that this very strip mall had been the scene of our first date.

"*Please,*" he said, and when I finally looked over, I was alarmed to see that he was crying.

I had never made anyone cry before. I thought one former boyfriend's head might explode when I dumped him the day after prom. We were still down the shore with friends at the time, stuck together in a small rental house on account of the rain. "Couldn't you do this *before* I paid for the prom tickets and the limo!?" he asked before stalking off to another room, leaving me to stew in the fact of my own horribleness. Another ex of mine eventually developed an ulcer after I broke up with him on five separate occasions—a reaction I thought was a bit excessive. In retrospect though, I *was* a pain. But this—the crying—was new.

"Michael. I'm just—I want to be able to see other people," I said. "I don't feel as if I can commit myself to one person right now." I looked back down at my hands. At my knuckles. At the pebbled surface of the steering wheel. Michael looked down into his lap and sighed. I sighed, too. Guilt blossomed and burned in my chest.

Still, I *had* tried to warn him. Months ago, when we first started dating, when he was still calling me at least once a day and already referring to me as "honey"— an endearment that made me feel twitchy in the way it seemed so proprietary—I told him straight-out what kind of person I was. At that point, I had become adept at shutting myself off from other people, at shrinking away before they could get close. And he was inching closer. As we pulled into the parking lot of my favorite all-night diner and slid out of the car, I slipped my warning easily enough into the conversation.

"You know, I'm not the kind of person you want as your girlfriend," I said. "You should know that now." I peered at him over the top of my car, catching his eye. "I feel as if monogamy is an unnatural societal construct, and I certainly don't believe in 'the one,'" I continued, shaking my head in dismissal. "After all, no one person can fulfill all of one's needs."

At the time, however, I didn't know Michael well. I didn't know that such a statement would only be seen as a personal challenge. By Michael's own admission years later, he liked to pursue difficult things.

And I certainly was difficult.

A month after I first declared to Michael my need for independence and autonomy, we had sex for the first time. Slowly, he had been inuring me to a life in which he played a leading role. We were spending almost every day together. On the days we didn't see each other, we spoke on the phone. And when we didn't do that, I missed him.

The day we first had sex was like most other days we spent together: we watched B-horror movies in bed, and then we let the intimacy of the setting take over. On this particular day, we watched *Rumpelstiltskin,* one of those old-fashioned flicks that is just the right amount of bad, allowing it to circle all the way back around to awesome. Hunchbacked gnomes, severed hands that could still give the finger, and catchy phrases like "This ain't no fairytale!"—it had it all. Afterward, we lay propped up against each other, so fully in each other's space that we had only to turn toward each other in order to find lips against lips, to share breath.

He stroked my bare arm and then leaned closer to cup one breast though my T-shirt. I arched toward him, pressed into him, the heat of his hand magnified by how much I wanted him. It was a feeling I hadn't experienced in quite some time, so preoccupied was I by pushing people away. But with him, the warmth spread across my skin, raised the hairs on my arms, made me jut my hips toward his.

Over the last couple months, I had relaxed into an ease with Michael in which I felt I could be completely myself. In past relationships I always felt I was playing an idealized version of myself—but also an unsustainable version of myself. This version lasted long enough for me to have fun, and then pull back, always leaving them wanting more. I never felt guilty about this because, for the most part, I assumed the men I was with were doing the same. But Michael always seemed so fully himself, even from the very beginning when he walked into my life wearing a frayed Pavement T-shirt with pictures of eggs over his nipples. From the beginning, he was goofy and unguarded and willing to say what he was thinking and feeling, even if it might be embarrassing. His willingness to be so openly imperfect made me feel that I could be the same. It made me feel safe. This, more than anything else, was sexy as hell.

We spent a good amount of time that day, post-*Rumpelstiltskin,* pressing our lips together, devouring each other between great gulps of air. Eventually, he undid the button on the fly of my jeans, pulled down the zipper, peeled my pants down the length of my legs and tossed them aside. He fumbled with his own shorts and then we wrestled together, rolling back and forth across the expanse of his mattress. When I landed on top, I hovered just above his boxer briefs, dipping my hips down and then rising up again and again, a slow torture. Finally, he raised his eyebrows at me, and I felt how the weight of my withholding had been suffocating me for so long. He pulled one leg hole of my cotton granny panties to the left and slid inside.

Later that afternoon, likely emboldened by his

success at finally consummating our relationship, he suggested we have sex again. This time, I wasn't so sure. I had spent so long holding back pieces of myself that it seemed wrong to let myself relax into full intimacy. And in the very back of my mind, sex was still very much bound up with fear and self-loathing. At the time, I didn't realize that my habitual guardedness was a natural reaction to the abusive relationship that had come before. It was only later that I would learn about how those who experience sexual and psychological abuse sometimes find connecting to others difficult. That they sometimes have difficulty with romantic intimacy, emotional connections, communication, and closeness. Sure, I suspected that my dearth of sexual desire had at its root that past sexual relationship. But I didn't know the ways in which those memories could be even more insidious, sabotaging any attempts at romantic connection I might make, physical or otherwise.

Having just kissed his way up my inner thighs, Michael knelt above me, leaned down for a kiss, and then rose up again. "Come on," he said, a slight smirk on his lips, being playful.

But suddenly, I no longer saw Michael hovering above me, legs straddling my torso. His smirk was a trip wire that took me back in time and, instead, I saw Travis, who never cared about what I wanted, or about what I wasn't ready for. I saw Travis's lips twisted into that smirk, cruel instead of playful. "Come on," he would say, pretending to tease me, begging for a blowjob or a quick dip into my panties. But really, he was impatient. He wanted me to be ready and willing to fulfill his every sexual want and need. And he always made me feel stupid for being scared.

With Michael still poised above me, waiting, I began to cry. "What's wrong?" he asked, clambering off me and reaching to touch my shoulder. I rolled away from him, drawing my knees in, and continued to cry, humiliated by my visceral reaction to an innocent phrase, an innocent smile. "What happened?" he asked.

And because I trusted him as I had trusted no one else in quite some time, I told him.

Opening myself up to Michael in such a big way did not magically cure me of my complicated relationship with sex, or with romantic and emotional intimacy. Over the coming weeks, I veered wildly between wanting that physical connection with him and not wanting sex at all. Somehow, Michael's steady patience and understanding only made it worse. I knew he deserved someone less damaged. Our relationship only served to confirm for me what I had suspected before: holding men at arm's length was what was best for both them and me.

Which is how we ended up in that Barnes & Noble parking lot, Michael knuckling away his tears while I looked away. "Listen," he said. "I don't want to stop seeing you. If you want to be able to see other people, we can do that. We can keep our relationship open."

"Michael—"

"I still want to be with you. Can you really say you don't care about me, too?"

I sighed again. No. I couldn't really say that.

Granted the dispensation to do whatever I wanted, thereby cementing my status as a woman who could not be pinned down, I began frequenting my local bar in order to flirt with other men. After all, as long as I was actively going out on dates with multiple dudes, my relationship with Michael could continue to be labeled as casual. So, on a stretch of highway outside town, where it shared a parking lot with a small, low-cost fitness center that held cardio kickboxing classes in the back room, the bar became my hunting ground for quick, superficial connection. I went there at least once a week with an old friend of mine, someone who didn't quite understand my inability to commit to Michael, but who was happy enough keeping an eye out for any eligible bachelors she might meet. Together, we sucked down mixed drinks through those tiny, plastic straws, swayed our hips to the latest cover band, and scanned the crowd for anyone who looked promising.

The pickings were decidedly slim.

After ending up in conversation with one guy, I teased him, telling him he looked and sounded like a car salesman. He pulled a crumpled business card out of the pocket of his jeans and passed it to me. It was for the Mazda dealership on Route 17 in Ramsey. We ended up in his car later on, leaning toward each other over the gear shift, his tongue pressing past my lips, cold from the beers he'd been drinking. Though the entire night had been leading to this, all I could think about was how different it all felt. How it lacked the heat of what I had with Michael. When my phone buzzed with texts from my friend wanting to know where the hell I was, I was almost relieved.

Another time, I ran into an old acquaintance from high school, someone I had always considered attractive, but who had been dating a friend of mine back then. We exchanged numbers and a week or so later I drove over to his house to pick him up for an ice cream date. As he slid into the passenger seat of my car, he glanced down at my white eyelet skirt. "Oh! You look like a nun!" he said, and I wasn't sure how to respond.

Later, stepping out of the car in the Carvel parking lot, he eyed my bare legs. "Ooh . . . a sexy nun," he corrected.

Yet another guy I met at the bar was a full foot taller than me. My friend's opening line was an astonished, "Gosh, you're tall!"

At the end of our first date, I was charmed when he said, "Well, this is the awkward moment when we decide whether or not to kiss!" And we did, hesitant and soft and chaste.

On our second date, suddenly conflicted by the ethics of juggling two men at once, I tried to explain The Status of My Romantic Life™. Tucked into a circular booth at Pizzeria Uno, I leaned across the table, my hands pressed flat on either side of my plate of pizza skins. "You should know that I'm seeing someone else," I said, afraid to look directly at him. "But we have an open relationship. We're both allowed to see other people."

He stared at me and I wiped a finger across the corner of my mouth, suddenly paranoid there might be sour cream on my face. "Huh," he finally said. "I don't know how to respond to that." The rest of the evening was awkward, filled with odd silences and a dearth of eye contact. I never heard from him again.

Meanwhile, as I was finally coming to remember how terrible dating really was, Michael and I continued to push and pull at each other, a dance that left each of us disgusted with each other one day and hungry for each other the next. And through it all, I couldn't help feeling frigid and unworthy of Michael's love.

By this point, I was working full-time for an academic book publisher, drawing up book contracts, proofreading back cover copy, and traveling to conferences. Though I loved the fact that I was working with books, I was disappointed that it didn't afford me the opportunity to write. I was moving around other people's words, but not putting together any of my own.

I sought out freelance work, armed only with a limited portfolio containing mostly porn and toy reviews from my college internship. To my surprise, I quickly learned that editors were eager for open, honest, and humorous sex writing. This was still a time, after all, when not every publication had its own resident sexpert. Even though I'd never aspired to be a career sex writer, I went all in. I became the books editor for a sex news site. I did volunteer publicity work for a magazine written by and for sex workers. I reviewed toys for AOL's now-defunct *Lemondrop* blog. I got my first print magazine clip in *Playgirl*.

Just as I had in college, I started to think of my sex writing as the thing that could fix my sex and relationship issues. *Maybe if I just try this*, I'd think, accepting an invitation to a sex party, *things between me and Michael will be easier. Maybe if I can successfully use this*, I'd think while reviewing a nice pair of handcuffs, *I can feel less lost in the bedroom. I can really let go.*

After a while, I couldn't help thinking that maybe it was working. Every so often, I would surprise myself with a sudden rush of desire, of physical need. Like that time after the Renaissance Faire when we climbed into my tiny twin bed, the both of us still covered in splotches of dirt from the mud show, pulling at brown-splattered T-shirts and sludge-stiff jeans. I pulled my cap-sleeved Ani DiFranco "ain't no damsel in distress" shirt up over my head and threw it to the other side of my room. Then I pulled him toward me, wrapping my legs around his torso, feeling his hip bones press sharply into my thighs. I kept pulling him in closer, deeper, despite knowing I'd find the bruises later on, scattered across the insides of my legs. They were like love bites, those marks, reminders that I was his.

And there was that time at a friend's house party, when Michael and I locked ourselves in her bedroom. We brought sleeping bags so we could stay over, but we both slithered into mine. Pressed so closely together, it didn't take much for him to pull my underpants out of the way and slip inside. When we heard her at the doorway, jiggling the knob, musing aloud as to why the heck the door was locked, we bucked against each other more quickly, finishing with a mutual gasp. By the time my friend got the door open, Michael was reclined casually in the sleeping bag and I was across the room, muttering about the beer I'd spilled on my shirt earlier in the evening.

But these quick bursts of intense physical connection didn't seem like enough to sustain a long-term relationship. And my frenzied purchases of bedroom how-to manuals and bullet vibrators weren't getting me any closer to sexual enlightenment. I knew that I loved Michael by this point, that I felt strange on the days I didn't see him. But the more he pushed me to surrender into full symbiosis with him, the more uncomfortable I felt accepting his love. I was still terrified of what an entire lifetime with Michael might look like, a lifetime during which I couldn't give him the amount of physical affection he deserved. I knew we would eventually grow to resent each other. He, because I couldn't give him the level of intimacy he wanted. I, because of the guilt and the pressure to perform. Obviously, we would resent each other. Maybe even come to hate each other. But it would be too late. We'd be stuck.

I asked myself: *If even his love can't fix me, can I be so sure he's really the one?*

I asked myself this question despite purportedly not believing in "the one." I was scared that the real reason I struggled to believe in the one was because I'd never experienced the blinding certainty of having met my soul mate. What if the person who could save me—who could fix me—was still out there? What if binding myself to Michael meant I could never be whole?

Our relationship collapsed over a weekend trip to Boston. During the four-hour drive to our hotel, we ran through all of the more delightful topics of conversation that were available to us until, inevitably, we ended up talking about the open nature of our partnership.

"You know, *you* can see other people, too," I said when Michael again pressed me to make our relationship monogamous. He'd been pressing for this ever since he'd agreed we could keep things non-monogamous.

"But I'm *not* seeing other people. I don't *want* to see other people," he said.

"But I do!" I said, glowering through the windshield

as we inched our way along the Mass Pike, my fingers cramping as I clenched the steering wheel. "And what you're *not* doing isn't the point. It's not like I'm keeping you from dating around. This was the deal we made." I glanced over at him as we made our excruciating way toward Boston. "If you didn't think you could handle it, you shouldn't have agreed to it!"

By the time we arrived at the hotel, we were barely speaking. Within fifteen minutes of checking into our room—wheeling in our suitcases, placing our toiletries in the bathroom, emptying our bladders—we had exploded into a full-on, scream-filled breakup. I stalked out of the room and called my mom, crying, from the hotel lobby. And then, because it had taken us four hours to drive there and because we had already committed to paying $170 a night to stay there for two nights, I stalked back upstairs and suggested we muddle our way through the weekend despite the circumstances.

Over the next few days, we power walked up and down the streets of Boston together, Michael trailing me as I strode ahead, my brow furrowed with equal parts anguish and purpose. We wandered the Boston Commons and the Public Garden, snapping photos of weeping willows and rose bushes and swan boats. We took the T out to Cambridge, walked the Harvard campus, browsed Newbury Comics where I bought candy apple red, heart-shaped sunglasses that I wore the rest of the weekend. We spent eighty minutes on one of the Duck Tours during which Michael leapt from his seat when they asked, in the middle of the Charles River, if there was anyone who wanted to steer the boat. (I'm pretty sure the offer was intended for the younger passengers.) We took selfies at the Christian Science Center reflecting pool, a spot I had always loved back when I was an undergrad at Emerson College, living just around the corner. Back then, the pool had been a place for quiet contemplation, or else it had been a place to meet up with friends, eating takeout cheesecake slices from the brand-new Cheesecake Factory. Now it was the site of my relationship's slow unraveling, its unending death rattle.

On the four-hour drive back to New Jersey, I set some ground rules. Due to the fact that we had managed to comport ourselves with dignity in the hours following our breakup, I sensed that Michael might be in a state of denial about the status of our relationship. And I was right.

"We had a great time together," he said. "Why would you still want to break up?"

I grinded my teeth together to keep from screaming. "We're already broken up," I said, enunciating each word carefully. "We made the best of a bad situation. But it's time to face reality." I took a breath. Let it out in an abrupt whoosh, my body deflating. "That fight we had," I reminded him. "Nothing has changed. The problems we've been having still exist. The things we've been fighting about are the same things we've been fighting about for weeks. If we stay together, we'll only keep fighting about them. Nothing will be resolved."

"But what about everything else?" he asked. "We're good together. You know we are."

"Michael!" I said, determined not to let him weaken my resolve for the second time, already feeling it weakening.

I sighed. I sighed a lot when I was around Michael.

"Listen," I said. "You need to at least give me some time. Some space. Time to think about what I want. Space to see what things are like without you."

He looked at me, pouting his lips, raising his hands in supplication, but I jumped in as he was opening his mouth to speak.

"No phone calls," I said. "No emails. No text messages. No messages of any sort."

He was quiet.

"I mean it," I said. "I need this."

He lasted just under two weeks. On a LiveJournal post in which I marveled that I had attended a networking event and ended up in an extended conversation with "The Most Attractive Guy to Ever Talk to Me Willingly," Michael commented, "silly girl, you know there is no man more attractive than me." Several weeks later, he sent me a birthday card emblazoned with a heart made of small, punched out circles. "I love you a hole punch," it said, and I shook my head and hung it up on the bulletin board behind my bedroom door.

Meanwhile, I tried to fill my days and evenings with writing, live music, beer, and books. I threw myself into work and went to networking events for publishing professionals. I edged my way back into the dating scene and went on Internet dates with guys who posted their ads on Nerve.com. Looking back from a remove of over fifteen years, I can't remember my exact state of mind where it concerns Michael, and my LiveJournal archives don't provide much in the way of clues. My mother, however, insists that I was a sobbing, sniveling mess, constantly second guessing my resolution to remove him from my life.

My mother's insistence on my alleged despair notwithstanding, what I do remember is that I missed him. After all, he had become such a part of my day to day that his absence made me feel as if things were just slightly off, like a picture on the wall that's been nudged askew. I had read once that to love someone is to miss them when they're not around. It was the type of quote you might stumble upon on Instagram, written out in a flowery font and surrounded by hearts and a curlicued border. But still. Did this not prove that what Michael and I shared was the real deal?

Looking back on all of the fights we ever had, none of them were really about him. All of them were about me. I'd spent the past four years pushing people away, not wanting any of them to get close enough to see the sexually dysfunctional mess I believed myself to be. If I let that happen, I'd then have to *explain* myself. It was a position of vulnerability I did not want to place myself in. I was scared that any man I explained myself to would think I was overreacting or making excuses. I was afraid they'd tell me to "get over it." I wished I could. I was already frustrated with myself and with my body for being unable to move past a six-month relationship that had occurred four flippin' years ago. If I never got close enough to anyone to actually get past third base, I could keep them from finding out how frigid I really was. Better to let the men who moved in and out of my life think I was fun and carefree and super-duper cool, and then cut them loose before they realized any different. Better to let them hear about the sex writing I'd done during college and make their own assumptions. Better to leave them wanting more.

Michael was the closest I'd ever come to revealing all of these parts of myself to someone else. And still, he wanted to be with me. This was terrifying, and I felt as if I were suffocating under the weight of his enduring affection. But even so, I missed him. What did that mean?

Almost two months after the separation I had imposed upon us, I began to waver. I agreed to hang out with Michael several times, in neutral environments that posed no danger of me, say, falling out of my underpants and into his bed. When Michael eventually asked me to be his girlfriend again, I said, "maybe." We both knew I meant "yes." What he didn't know was that this was a huge gamble for me. I was taking the risk that someday he'd become frustrated by all the things that didn't come easily to me and decide I wasn't worth loving. It drove me crazy that I couldn't be certain this wouldn't happen. But I was starting to suspect I would never be certain. And I didn't know if I could spend the rest of my life alone. Someday, I wanted a family.

Three months after getting back together, on a lower Manhattan sidewalk filled with a river of people dressed up as Santa Claus, in the midst of the chaos that is Santacon, Michael asked me to be his Mrs. Claus. "You're *weird*," I said, because I thought he was kidding.

But then Michael pulled us off to the side so the other Santas could move past us, and he wrestled a pale gray, velvet box out of the depths of his giant red Santa pants and held it out to me. I immediately recognized it as the box for my great-great-grandmother's engagement ring.

This is happening, I thought to myself as I breathed in the scent of sweat and liquor and candy canes, the cold winter air hitting the back of my throat. My cheeks and the tip of my nose were numb, and I shivered as I eyeballed the tiny box. *This is happening,* I told myself again, though I still didn't quite believe it. Michael flipped the lid open, I pulled my gloves off with my teeth, and he slid the ring onto my finger. "Okay," I said, looking down at the tier of diamonds sparkling in the cold, glaring light of December, still not sure how to feel. I looked back up at him. "Okay."

At the same time that I was coming to know Michael, moving in slow motion toward the day when I would eventually agree to commit myself to him and only him, I was simultaneously building a relationship with the only therapist I've ever loved. Though she wasn't a certified sex therapist—a specialization I could probably have benefited from—she was proving herself to be the perfect person to support me in my struggles with chronic depression and anxiety, issues I had been dealing with for years, even before my time with Travis. And so, I unloaded upon her all of my tales of professional and relationship angst without ever delving too deeply into what had happened with Travis all those years ago and how it still affected me. Part of me didn't want to admit that I was still dealing with the echoes of that relationship. Besides, I had plenty of other neuroses to keep the two of us occupied indefinitely.

When I look back now on all the years I spent seeing Dr. Jill, I see immediately that the topic of all of our conversations can be boiled down to a single concern: fear of making the wrong decision, and of then being stuck with the consequences of that terrible decision.

This fear manifested itself in my career choices. It manifested in the way I made plans to attend or not attend events that might set off my anxiety. It manifested in the way I had grappled with—and continued to grapple with—the question of whether or not to commit fully to spending the rest of my life with Michael. Even after saying "yes" to Michael's proposal, I was still afraid I had made the wrong choice.

Dr. Jill wasn't there when I was twenty, when I had finally gathered the strength to leave Travis but afterward had nothing left. She wasn't there when I eventually found that the only way to really move past everything was to flee, to drop out of school, to move four hours away to Boston.

Dr. Jill wasn't there when I was twenty-three, working as an editor at the environmental engineering firm, sometimes closing myself into an abandoned corner office, sitting on the windowsill, wondering if I was brave enough to pitch myself out into the open air.

Dr. Jill wasn't there when I was twenty-four, only a few weeks into a new job when I had a panic attack, and with my heart scrabbling its way up my throat, I quietly gathered my things and walked out, never to return. I remember emailing my former boss later that night and, the next morning, ignoring the ringing of the telephone as she left message after message.

But Dr. Jill knew all of these stories. She could see my restlessness in my relationship and in my present job and understand it for what it was.

"How can you feel motivated," she once asked me, "if you can't see your future?"

And: "Think back to all of those places in which you felt stuck. The unhealthy relationship. The job. Are you still there?"

"No," I would whimper sheepishly.

"Then were you ever really stuck?"

Seeing Dr. Jill became the highlight of my week. On Wednesdays, at the end of the work day, I would shrug on my coat and sling my bag over my shoulder and take the elevator down to the lobby and burst out into daylight and, already, I would feel my entire body humming in anticipation. I would walk the nineteen blocks down toward the Flatiron Building—which always seemed to glow on sunny days—and the one block over, and I would enter the office building where my therapist saw her clients and, when she opened her door to me and smiled, I would feel relief.

After the marriage proposal, I talked to Dr. Jill about how I was afraid of committing myself to one person for the rest of my life. How I was afraid I would ruin everything.

"People always say that they knew they'd found 'the one,'" I said to Dr. Jill. "I don't feel that sense of certainty. Does that mean that this is all a huge mistake?"

Dr. Jill didn't tell me that these were normal, pre-wedding jitters. She didn't rush to reassure me, didn't tell me that Michael and I were meant for each other, that our marriage would be a glorious, glowing success, that we would ride off into the sunset together on a wave of rainbows and scented confetti. After all, I couldn't expect Dr. Jill to make my decision for me: bestowing upon me her blessing or advising me to flee. That was a risk I had to take myself. Instead, Dr. Jill responded in the way she always responded to my irrational fears over the things I could not possibly control or foresee. "You're not stuck if it doesn't work out," she said. "He can always leave you. You can always leave him." It wasn't romantic, but it was certainly level-headed.

We also talked a bit about my lackluster sex life, dampened especially by the emergence of pain during intercourse. After an initial few months in which I had wanted Michael, wanted to sleep with him as often as possible, our relationship had lapsed into that place where, once again, sex was a struggle for me. "Well of course you're never in the mood for sex," she said. "Why would you look forward to it if you were only anticipating that it would hurt?"

It could be that, because of Dr. Jill's lack of training in the area of sexuality, she would never have been able to draw the line from my relationship with Travis to my continuing depression, the panic attacks, the fear. Or it could be that she never realized the extent of the impact he'd had on my life because I minimized it too much.

I've since learned that women who have been sexually assaulted have a greater chance of experiencing PTSD, anxiety, and depression and, by extension, sexual dysfunctions like dyspareunia (one of the possible diagnoses when one experiences pain during intercourse). I've learned that my difficulties with romantic intimacy, my struggle to let others—to let Michael—get close, are common. Intimacy, after all, becomes associated with danger. Those who have experienced sexual assault or other forms of intimate partner violence often avoid sexual intimacy, which can then lead to strain in later romantic relationships.

But when I was seeing Dr. Jill, neither of us made those connections. I didn't talk about Travis very often. Though my sex writing had been motivated by a desire to move past the effects of our relationship, I still didn't realize the full force of the impact he'd had. His power. I didn't want to see that particular truth.

"Were you ever really stuck?" asked Dr. Jill, with the implication that I never really could be.

But marriage was supposed to be forever. That was the definition of stuck.

On the day Michael asked me to be his Mrs. Claus—ring box held out in his red, wind-chapped hands and I in a mild state of shock—I was finally forced to make a decision. One I had been waffling on for the past year and a half.

At that point in my life, what I wanted more than anything else was to be normal. I wanted to be in a romantic relationship in which I wasn't always looking over my shoulder for the exit sign. I wanted to have a sex life that wasn't so fraught. One in which I experienced desire that was equal to that of my partner's, in which I didn't feel inferior, in which I didn't hurt. I wanted to know love. To know it *was* love, without doubt. I wanted to someday walk down an aisle, say "I do," so I could then buy a house with bay windows and a kitchen island and a sun room and built-in bookshelves.

I wanted to be a mother.

Many of these things hadn't happened for me yet with Michael. I was still hedging my bets. Keeping an eye on that exit sign. I was experiencing dramatic dips in sexual desire. Feeling pain in bed. I knew I loved Michael. Yes. But was I *in* love?

Still, when I was with Michael, I felt safe. When I was with Michael, I felt comfortable. When I looked at Michael, I saw the father he could someday be.

When I looked at Michael, I could see a future.

I had never seen a future with anyone else. And so, when he held out that ring box, when he asked me to be his Mrs. Claus as I stood there with hundreds of other Santas rushing by me in an unending wave, the wind at my back, the sun in my eyes, I took a breath and said, "okay."

4 | PRETENDING TO BE THE COOL GIRL

I was at a cocktail party for people working in tech when I ended up in conversation with a random web developer. We were at a bar in east Midtown filled with a mix of web developers in ill-fitting button-downs, pit stains expanding toward rib cages, and a smattering of female bloggers. We were all sardined together, pushed up against the curve of the bar, pushing between each other to get from one end of the room to the other. Our gazes slid automatically down toward each other's breast bones, as tends to happen at events where the measure of your worth can be found in black magic marker on your self-adhesive name tag. A mix of sweat, B.O., and various colognes hung in the air and scrabbled its way down my throat. The web developer and I ended up next to each other, shoulders rammed together, as we both tried to make eye contact with the bartender, free-drink tickets growing damp in our hands.

"Sorry," I muttered, though it was no one's fault we were invading each other's personal space.

He shrugged, forcefully angled his body toward me,

looked at my chest, squinted his eyes. "YourTango . . .?" he asked, reading aloud from my name tag. "What's that?"

And that's how we ended up talking about the fact that I was a sex writer, working as a perma-lance editor at an online magazine that published content on love and relationships.

We remained pressed together like that for almost an hour. He may have even bought me a drink or two, large glasses of Pinot Grigio that allowed me to feel looser in my skin, less tense as the taste of acid and grape-fruit worked their way across my tongue and down my esophagus. He peppered me with questions about the work I did and, eventually, I lost track of the person I arrived with.

As the hour grew late, I felt my energy plummet in one quick whoomp, and I looked toward the front door, a sea of elbows and hip bones and straining stomachs separating us.

"I should probably head home," I said, looking point-edly at the time on my cell phone, pulling a cardigan out of my bag. After determining that we were both going to the Port Authority, he offered to walk with me.

We were mostly quiet as we walked west. I was lost in thought, trying to gauge which bus I might catch. As we stepped off the curb to cross another avenue, he took my hand, presumptuously, I thought, as if to keep me safe. He didn't let go when we'd reached the other side, and I didn't pull away. I didn't want to insult him. He must have felt the stones on my wedding band and engagement ring digging into the undersides of his fingers. But he didn't seem to care.

"You know, hearing about your work really turns me on," he said as we walked the last block before Eighth Avenue, and my stomach lurched.

I pulled my hand away then, digging in my purse for nothing. "Even sex gets boring," I said, trying to sound breezy, trying to defuse whatever it was he was feeling, whatever it was he thought I had invited by admitting to being a sex writer. I was relieved when we entered the Port Authority, the overhead lights seeming to create a new distance between us. The late-night commuters, the drunks, the shambling homeless made me feel safe.

He wanted to find a quiet corner where we could be alone together. He kept insisting. Instead of telling him he had no right to assume I would do anything with him, I made some excuse about the bus schedule. I didn't want to cause a scene. I didn't want to seem uptight. When he finally turned away, disappointed and defeated, and descended down an escalator, I let my breath out in a gasp. Once he was out of sight, I turned and walked briskly to my gate, almost at a jog. The back of my neck felt hot and prickly, as if I suspected he may have changed his mind and followed me.

Being a sex writer has always made me unsure of how I'm supposed to be. Wild? Daring? Brazen? Nonchalant? It has made me unsure of how I'm supposed to feel. Of whether or not I should maybe want it—sex— more. Of where the line might be between harmless banter within the context of work that already includes sex, and sexual harassment. *Am I too sensitive?* I often wonder to myself. *Too vanilla? Too much of a prude?*

My first employer in the world of sex writing was always pressing up against these boundaries. He openly speculated about what his female employees might be like in bed. He gave unsolicited lectures about the logistics of anal beads. Because of my willingness to test out all manner of vibrators, he referred to me as the Vibrator Queen.

Sometimes I decided maybe this was appropriate workplace repartee, considering the fact that we were developing content for an adult personals site. Again, there was that fear of being seen as uptight . Deep down, however, I knew it wasn't okay. I knew that the longer I let things to continue in this manner—the longer I kept my mouth shut and allowed the boundary between professional and personal to blur—the more I was essentially consenting to his behavior. Or, considering that this was in the days before "yes means yes" became a feminist rallying cry, that's how he might interpret it.

One of the last times we were in contact was when I accompanied him on a day trip to Philadelphia for a publishing conference. Michael had recently proposed to me and, as I waited with my boss for our train ride back home, we discussed the likelihood that my marriage would stand the test of time.

"It's never going to work," he said, as if he could see the future and know, without a doubt, that the demise of my marriage was an inevitability. My face prickled with heat, and my stomach lurched. It was if he had looked into my very soul and seen all my doubts, all the ways in which I'd imagined us falling apart.

"Why?" I asked him, trying to conjure up a bravado I didn't actually feel. "Why wouldn't it work?"

"Because you need strange cock," he said, as if he knew anything at all about my sex life—which he didn't.

He didn't even know that I'd been scared of sex when he first met me several years before, interviewing me and hiring me to write adult content. He didn't know that I was still scared of it. He didn't know that I was unable to enjoy it, and that I was only writing about it to fix that part of me that seemed broken. He didn't know anything about the real me at all, because I hadn't shown him.

Even though it wasn't my responsibility to educate him about appropriate boundaries, I still worried that his behavior toward me was my own fault. After all, I had laughed along at the office even when it felt uncomfortable. I had shown unending tolerance.

Travis had made me self-conscious about my lack of experience in the bedroom, and I didn't want to be the person that Travis had known. I didn't want to be that shrinking, tedious person he made me feel I was. So, just as I'd done years ago in the moment that eventually led me to write about sex in the first place, I never said "no" or "stop" to my employer either.

After my initial stint with sex writing, none of my subsequent employers ever spoke to me in the crude manner my first employer had, even though the focus of my work continued to be sex. They knew better. They maintained a higher level of professionalism and maturity around the topic of sex, with the mentality that sex writing was no different from any other career path one might choose for oneself.

But I did receive an interesting mix of reactions when I told new acquaintances what I did for a living. Like the tech nerd at the bar, for example. The presumptuous one. He wasn't the only man who assumed that because

I wrote about sex, I must be some sort of sex maniac who was always up for a tumble in the hay.

Other men assumed I was a sex pro, master of every position in the Kama Sutra, able to perform amazing feats of lovemaking that would automatically make any partner scream with pleasure. This assumption made me nervous, as it couldn't be further from the truth. And it was especially problematic when it came from someone with whom I was trying to build a relationship (in the days before I met my husband, of course). I often found myself resisting intimacy with these men because I was embarrassed by what they would discover once the clothes came off. My awkwardness. My ineptitude. My disquieting levels of silence while doing the deed. Knowing a lot about sex did not make me good at it. And because I was so afraid of being a massive disappointment in bed, these relationships were doomed from the start.

Perhaps the primary reason things worked out so well with Michael is because I was on hiatus from sex writing when we first met, and I was still on hiatus when we eventually began sleeping together. Later on in our relationship, after I had returned to writing about sex on the regular, he basked in the bad-ass cred my sex writing career gave him as someone who was allegedly married to a nymphomaniacal sexpert. But he never had any of the expectations other men did. He knew better.

The response I faced from women was more varied, and sometimes more complex. For the most part, the knowledge that I was a sex writer made women want to confide in me, talk about their own struggles, gain assurance from me that they were "normal." That their marriage was normal. That what they were experiencing was normal. They told me things I'm sure they never felt comfortable telling their primary care physicians or their gynecologists or even their partners.

Some women asked if I could recommend resources for mismatched libidos or lackluster marital sex, revealing things about their intimate lives they likely would not have divulged otherwise. I told them what I had learned or pointed them toward content I had already published. Much of the time, however, having a nonjudgmental person listen to them—someone who wouldn't bat an eye at mid-intercourse queefing, or low sexual frequency, or chronic vaginal dryness—was all they needed.

Other women—a small subset—seemed to feel defensive when faced with the details of my career. Maybe they, too, assumed I was a pro in the bedroom, the real-life embodiment of their partners' sexual fantasies. Maybe they saw me as a threat because they, like me, were harboring doubts about their abilities in the bedroom. "I never needed all those bells and whistles," they would say with a snarl in their voice when I explained that I used to review vibrators and vibrating cock rings and erotic films. Like they were better than that and, by extension, better than me. Deep down, I worried they were.

Some women were flustered or embarrassed by my job, leading me to lean into flippancy and then change the subject. Some were fascinated and wanted to know more. In time, I learned to alter my response to the question *What do you do?* depending upon who was doing the asking. "I'm a sex writer" or "I write about sex"

I would say straight-out if I sensed the person could handle it. Sometimes I would just say, "I'm a writer."

When I was invariably asked what I wrote about, I would say "sexual health" or "female sexuality" or "health and wellness" because these phrases seemed less frivolous. Less dirty. More legitimate, connected as they were to the unquestionable authority of the medical field. You see, one must be extremely calculating when talking about sex, no matter who's in the audience. This is one thing I learned.

I also learned that the virgin/whore complex is still alive and well and is only amplified when you write about sex for a living.

Journalist Rachel Hills recently discussed this double bind women are in regarding their sexuality in her book *The Sex Myth: The Gap Between Our Fantasies and Reality* (2014). Hills acknowledges the enduring attitude in our culture that we are dirty if we have too much sex. She then argues that, in our sex-saturated culture, we are simultaneously considered frigid, or even deficient, if we don't have *enough* sex.

After all, in our culture of tell-all memoirs (*Whip Smart, The Sexual Life of Catherine M., Secret Diary of a Call Girl*) and sex-focused TV shows and movies (*Masters of Sex, Californication, Nymphomaniac*), and with a different online sexpert or confessional writer baring all at every publication you might click over to, who wants to admit they're only having sex once a week, or that they've never gone shopping at Babeland or Good Vibrations, or that their favorite position is missionary?

At the same time, god forbid you admit that you

masturbate or enjoy sex or *maaaaaybe* spend a bit too much time searching the Internet for audio porn. Good girls don't do that, as is evidenced by the fates of female protagonists in such pop cultural touchstones as *The Virgin Suicides, Jennifer's Body, Teeth,* and *Twilight.* On the one hand, we have sexually voracious women being equated with demonic succubae. On the other hand, we have young women who are glorified for their purity, and then viciously punished when they stray.

We see this in the real-life criticism women receive when they revel in their bodies (Kim Kardashian "breaking the Internet" with her butt or Beyoncé being tsk-tsk'd after being photographed in her underwear) or embrace their sexuality (the slut-shaming of pop stars such as Miley Cyrus and Britney Spears when they broke out of their confining Disney boxes).

Where does that leave someone like me who is neither a paragon of purity, nor a true sexual omnivore? How do I sustain a dialogue about sexuality when I am not the sexual being people expect me to be?

Ariel Levy touched upon this trend of simultaneously praising and punishing sexuality years before Hills in her 2006 book *Female Chauvinist Pigs: Women and the Rise of Raunch Culture*. In it, she writes about women who embrace their sexuality as an emblem of their empowerment, trying to be one of the guys while simultaneously being the girl those guys would like to fuck.

This characterization is echoed in the concept of the "Cool Girl"—that embodiment of womanhood recently made popular by Gillian Flynn's character Amy Dunne in *Gone Girl*. In her journal, Amy writes that:

> Being the Cool Girl means I am a hot, brilliant, funny woman who adores football, poker, dirty jokes, and burping, who plays video games, drinks cheap beer, loves threesomes and anal sex, and jams hot dogs and hamburgers into her mouth like she's hosting the world's biggest culinary gang bang while somehow maintaining a size 2, because Cool Girls are above all hot. Hot and understanding. Cool Girls never get angry; they only smile in a chagrined, loving manner and let their men do whatever they want. (Dunne, pp. 222-223)

I remember feeling a click of recognition upon reading the "Cool Girl" passage in *Gone Girl*, accompanied by a frisson of resentment. After all, isn't that the part I play every time I explain my job to anyone, man or woman? Because who wants to hear about the reality? Who wants to hear about all the sex I'd rather not be having and all the ways in which both our culture and the pharmaceutical industry are conspiring to make me feel like shit because of it? My favorite vibrator or my most highly recommended personal lubricant may not be considered TMI, but *that* bit of hard reality certainly is.

Most of the people willing to talk to me about their own uninspiring sex lives are the ones who already know my story. Or the ones who have read my story online and have commented or emailed me, thanking me for my honesty because now they know they are not alone. The words I share give them the permission they need to admit that, like me, they're not having the amount of sex or the type of sex they're made to feel they should be having.

I've received similarly mixed messages in the work I've done. One of the sex columns I wrote was never featured on the site's home page because the publishers didn't want to scare off advertisers. So . . . sex sells, but it doesn't sell ads. Another site, whose entire identity (and subsequent popularity) was based around an open honesty and explicitness about sex, rebranded itself as a general lifestyle site. It seems that the grasping for dwindling advertising dollars beginning to mark online publishing superseded the site's desire to maintain their unique identity and retain their original audience.

More recently, *Playboy,* of all publications, announced that they would no longer be printing nudes in their pages (though they later flip-flopped on this decision). With these decisions, these publications have made themselves indistinguishable from all of the other "lifestyle" sites that are courting sexy content without committing to it. In this, the publishing world is like a microcosm of culture at large: filled with people who want to appear edgy, but who are simultaneously afraid of offending people's delicate sensibilities.

But who am I to chastise them for their prudish ways? I'm the biggest prude of all! I am a sex writer who does not want sex. And the fact that the person people assume me to be is so far removed from the person I actually am only adds to my feelings of shame and inferiority and full-blown impostor syndrome.

The assumptions people make about me—and the ways in which they sexualize me against my will—continue to make me uncomfortable. I still remember the very first time it happened, after I reviewed the Sexerciseball for AOL's *Lemondrop* blog. The

Sexerciseball was a large, blow-up exercise ball with a built-in adapter for the several dildos that came with it. I tried it while my husband was at work, using a pump to blow it up in our living room, flipping the blinds closed, twirling on the most basic dildo attachment, and sliding on a lubricated condom. I slapped on large quantities of additional lube for good measure and balanced myself awkwardly over the dildo, able to slide the entire length of it inside pretty easily, my inner thighs squealing against the rubber of the ball. I even bounced up and down a few times. But mostly, I was nervous I might lose my balance and start rolling across the living room, the dildo still inside me.

Which is exactly what I wrote when I did my review for *Lemondrop*, a post that was far more slapstick than sexy. But still, among the handful of comments the post received was one that made me feel decidedly uncomfortable:

Is it strange to admit that your awkwardness in this review turned me on?

It was the first comment I'd ever received that made me feel objectified, but it wouldn't be the last.

What feels like more of a betrayal, however, are the comments I sometimes receive from friends and family, the assumptions they make about me because of the things I write. Once at my in-laws' house, with relatives visiting from out of town, my mother-in-law made a joke about sex. "But I hear my daughter-in-law knows all about that kind of stuff," she sniggered. I blushed, feeling humiliated, feeling like the butt of a joke, because that's what she made me out to be. I know that such comments are likely motivated by discomfort with what I write about and aren't meant with malicious intent, but it feels hurtful to receive subtle slut jokes when what I write is important to me. At the same time, it feels disorienting to know that I am nothing like the sex writer people assume me to be. Again, I don't know how to feel. I don't know how to be.

Which is why, when my unassuming tech nerd from that cocktail party made me feel all squicky by presuming we would mess around, I hesitated to tell him off. "I don't want to miss my bus," I said, shrugging off the larger implications of our conversation. "I'm feeling a little tired and I don't want to get home too late," I added, as if I might have let him touch me if only circumstances had been different. "I'm in a monogamous relationship," I said, "and I don't think he'd be too thrilled." As if my husband's traditional approach to marriage was the problem.

What I didn't say . . . what I should have said, was: "I don't want to fool around, and I think it's presumptuous of you to assume I would just because of the work I do. Just because we had a friendly conversation. Just because we walked to the Port Authority together."

I didn't say it because I was still playing my part. I was still pretending to be the Cool Girl, the one who didn't blink an eye at innuendo, the one you might possibly get lucky with if all of the stars aligned just right.

I didn't say it because, despite my experience with Travis, I still believed most men would wait for my "yes" instead of barreling forward when they didn't hear a "no."

I believed this despite knowing that men already

assumed I had given my consent just by dint of being someone who spoke and wrote openly about sex. I believed this despite knowing that my writing resumé was the professional equivalent of a short skirt and a tight top, or a few too many drinks. I believed this despite knowing that the sexualization of sexuality professionals is a common issue in the field, so much so that presentations are sometimes given on the topic at professional sexuality conferences, and that academic papers exist on the objectification of sexuality researchers.[2]

The first time I attended the National Sex Ed Conference, a four-day sex educator conference in Atlantic City, New Jersey, I felt drawn to attend a workshop on the sexualization of sex educators. Even though I was there covering the conference for several different publications, gathering information on peer-to-peer sex ed programs and issues of cultural competency, that workshop felt particularly relevant to my interests. So I crept into the spacious room where the session was being held, with its wall of windows looking out over the Atlantic City beach, and found myself a seat near the back. As the rows of chairs began to fill up, I looked around at my fellow attendees. There were educators, yes, but there were also clinicians and researchers and program coordinators and nurses. Despite the variety, as the lone writer at the conference, I felt a bit out of place.

---

2   E. L. Zurbriggen. "II. Sexual Objectification by Research Participants: Recent Experiences and Strategies for Coping." Feminism & Psychology 12, no. 2 (2002): 261-68. doi:10.1177/095 9353502012002014.

As the session began, the co-facilitators immediately got attendees involved, asking them to shout out the types of people they'd been sexualized by so they could write all of the answers on a giant easel pad at the front of the room.

"My students!" shouted one woman, and it was written down in bright blue marker on the pad of paper.

"Prospective partners!" shouted another and this, too, was added as we all nodded our heads in recognition.

"And present partners," pointed out another.

"Mmmhmm . . ." I heard from somewhere else in the room.

"Colleagues," came a voice from the very back of the room, and we all whipped our heads around. The woman writing down all of our answers struggled to keep up.

"Sexual health colleagues or others?" asked the other facilitator.

"Both!" shouted someone else, and they were both added to the paper.

"Family members," said someone else, and I swallowed hard. I could feel a pressure building behind my eyeballs, and I felt as if I hadn't stopped nodding since we started.

"Complete strangers," said another, and I thought back on the many incidents from the past fifteen years.

"Everyone," said someone else, and the woman at the front of the room added it to the list, writing the word in all capital letters. As she wrote down the E, the V, the next E, and onward, each letter was like a fist squeezing my heart until I could feel my heartbeat throbbing in my throat.

I had felt like an outsider at the conference up until then, not being a certified sexuality professional myself. In that moment, however, I belonged. I had never before felt so fully understood.

Even having experienced that sense of belonging, however, it is still difficult to know how to respond when others make inappropriate comments. There is still that desire to make the *other* person feel comfortable and at ease. Even when it's someone I know. Even when it's someone I love.

And if I feel that way now, even after all I've learned, you can bet your ass that I was feeling that same sense of caution and trepidation when I met that delightful tech guy way back in the day at that ill-fated networking event.

Back then, I skirted the issue and avoided calling him out on his inappropriate behavior because I believed I was protecting myself. I had come to know that women can't prioritize their own sense of comfort and self-agency without forfeiting their safety.

But in protecting myself, what was I giving up?

5 | OUR LIFE AS AN EXPERIMENT

I was twenty when I finally succumbed to Travis's appeals for a blowjob. We had just shared a shower and I was feeling generous, so I knelt down on the bathroom floor as he stood before me, the hair on his legs dripping, making golden loops and whorls across his shins and down his calves. The mirror over the sink was fogged, and the air was damp and heavy. My knees were slick, tender as they dug into the tiled floor; wet strands of hair striped my cheeks and my forehead and inched between my lips, requiring me to spit them out before returning to the job at hand. Travis's knees shook, and he gasped. "Where did you learn to do that?" he asked.

Back when I still lived with my parents, I sometimes watched fuzzed-out porn at three in the morning. I stared at bodies twisting and humping on the screen, squinting to get a glimpse of things I'd not yet experienced. What was taking place on that bathroom floor was not nearly as *bow-chik-a-bow-wow* as what I had seen on TV. But as for sex education, that was all I had to go on. Apparently, it was enough.

You should never, however, underestimate the sex toy industry's ability to make you doubt yourself. Like a SkyMall for sexy time, adult toy developers love creating unnecessary doo-dads and whatzits that promise to elevate the in-and-out experience.

The BlowGuard was one such whatzit. Years after that first blowjob, when I received a review unit just before a romantic anniversary trip to a B&B in upstate New York, I slipped it into my suitcase. In the fullness of that first day upstate, I almost forgot about it. Leaving our luggage at the inn, we drove along the Canandaigua wine trail, turning in at small vineyards, poring over lists of whites and reds, swirling the wine in our glasses as if we knew what we were doing. We sipped Chambourcins and Sauvignon Blancs and Pinot Noirs and, later in the evening, gulped down large, full glasses of wine at the farm-to-table restaurant where we had our dinner. By the time we made our way back to our room, we were thoroughly soused. Especially Michael. Because my tolerance for alcohol was lower than his, I often used his glass as a personal dump bucket when we were at tastings.

A drunk Michael is a particularly frisky Michael. So as I bent over the sink in our private bathroom, brushing my teeth, he took the opportunity to remove all of his clothing except for his boxer briefs, clamber up onto the elevated canopy bed, and stretch out in a come-hither position. I looked at him when I emerged from the bathroom and shook my head. I was wearing bulky, fleece pajama pants emblazoned with a Cookie Monster pattern. We were still in our twenties, but we had never been what I'd describe as sexy. At least not in that performative way you see on TV and in the movies where the woman shimmies out of her negligee or the man backs his partner against the wall, and then they both magically orgasm while they're still standing there, dry humping each other. But I did have *one* ace up my sleeve.

I whipped the BlowGuard out of my suitcase and brandished it in the air. "Ta-daaaaa!"

Michael sighed.

The BlowGuard was a toy meant to be used during partner play in order to prevent you from nicking your partner with your teeth during oral sex. With its built-in bullet vibrator, it also promised "mind-blowing" pleasure. It looked like a mouth guard but, since we weren't winning points for sexiness anyway, I was willing to look silly if it meant we would soon experience staggering levels of orgasmic bliss.

The first speed bump came when I couldn't fit the bullet vibe into the dental guard. Michael grappled with it for a while before finally prevailing over imperfect manufacturing. Then, I realized I wasn't sure whether I was supposed to place the BlowGuard over my upper or lower teeth. The instructions that came with the device were less than illuminating.

I eventually decided to try it both ways (I am nothing if not thorough) but couldn't stop myself from giggling as I slow-motion approached my husband's penis.

Not only that, but I couldn't stop worrying that the BlowGuard would fall out of my mouth. This thought made me tense my jaw, which in turn made me worry that teeth nicks were inevitable. My tightened jaw also made it impossible for me to actually fit my husband's penis into my mouth. (He asserts that this is because his member is so large.)

Finally, we were forced to abort the experiment.

"Besides," he said, "it's scary to see that thing coming at my penis."

Luckily, we were able to laugh about it. But it wasn't always that way. When Michael and I weren't laughing, I was crying, the guilt and pressure I felt around my sexual issues suffocating me. If it were up to Michael, we would probably have sex every damn day. But night after night, when he turned to me in bed to run a hand down my arm, I turned away from him and stuck my head in a book. The want I'd felt for him at the beginning of our relationship had faded, and I could go for long stretches of time without feeling that tingling sensation that signified my desire. At the time, I hadn't yet learned that, for many women, physical arousal is the thing that *sparks* desire. I hadn't yet learned about the waxing and waning of desire that is normal throughout the course of everyone's life. And so, I resented him for pushing me, even after I told him I wasn't in the mood.

All of this was made worse by the fact that I continued to experience pain during intercourse for several years. Lube didn't help. Penetration wasn't the problem. It was when he was inside me, thrusting his way to completion, that I felt a sharp, stinging agony, like needles biting into my vaginal walls. Why would I want to participate in *that*? How could I not resent the person who wanted to forge ahead anyway, despite knowing what I was being forced to endure?

At the same time, I always felt that he deserved more. Better. And my experimentation around sex toys and my immersion in the world of sex positivity—an exploration enabled by my sex writing—were the vehicles I had chosen in my efforts to fix myself. I wanted to be more like everyone else. I wanted to have the sex life I imagined everyone else was having. I wanted to want. I wanted to feel comfortable and capable in bed. And if the pain I felt was all in my head—as my gynecologist at one point intimated—I wanted to get down to the very essence of who I was, deep down inside, and fix that, too.

When I first met Michael, it had been a little over a year since I'd written about sex within the context of my internship . . . and about the same amount of time since I'd had it. The latter situation soon changed. After connecting on Friendster, Internet stalking each other on LiveJournal, and courting each other via email (this sentence makes me feel ancient), we met IRL at a strip mall Dunkin' Donuts that was equidistant between our two homes. The connection between us was fairly instant and easy, and we proceeded to see each other every single day that first week. We became intimate within our first couple months of dating.

But it was at least another year before I found my way back to sex writing. And until that happened, I continued to feel lost in the bedroom, inadequate because of my low libido and desperate to find the thing that would boost my sex drive. Not for myself, but for Michael. Not so I could enjoy sex more, but so I could satisfy the man I was growing to love. So I could be the woman he deserved.

It was during this time I decided to interview a sex

party hostess as a means of getting her opinion for a class assignment on what Ariel Levy referred to as "raunch culture." When this popular party hostess invited me to her next sexy soiree, I grasped at the opportunity. "This will be so good for us!" I told Michael as I begged him to accompany me to the party.

I saw this sex party as my entrée back into a world in which I could use my sex writing credentials as a means of exposing both myself and my partner to experiences that would challenge me sexually. Also, as adventurous as sex writing would in time force me to be, there was no way in hell I was attending my very first orgy alone.

The first party we attended together was the best party, probably because neither of us had any particular expectations for the evening ahead of us. Instead, we felt a mixture of awkward and anxious and curious, and just a little bit excited.

Due to the novelty of this particular occasion, I decided it was best to plan ahead. First, I pulled the most revealing articles of clothing out of my closet, mixing and matching tank tops and skirts and pants, trying to find just the right combination of understated eroticism. Michael, meanwhile, dirty danced around our bedroom wearing black sweatpants and a black bow tie, the pallid skin of his chest and the xylophone of his ribs glowing in the harsh glare of the overhead light. He looked like a pale, scrawny Chippendales dancer. "How's this look?" he asked, licking his lips with mock sensuousness.

I crossed my arms across my chest. "Nope."

Next, I packed my bag. I crammed my wallet, a tube of tinted lip gloss, and a bottle of cheap wine into a floppy tote. I added in a variety pack of condoms, my favorite vibrator, and a pair of leather handcuffs. I didn't know what to expect from the evening ahead, so I wanted to be prepared for any eventuality. What if people got naked as soon as they stepped through the door? What if I was propositioned by someone who was into BDSM? What if we walked in on a giant orgy and my clitoris wasn't in the mood to come out and play? My tiny vibrator might mean the crucial difference between smoking hot sex play and a big fat raspberry of a disappointing time.

When it was finally time to head into Manhattan, we left our car in a secluded section of our suburban New Jersey town, taking a bus that ran long and local before finally reaching the lead-up to the Lincoln Tunnel. After arriving in the city, we power walked our way south about ten or fifteen blocks, my overstuffed bag slamming against my right thigh the entire way. As we approached the Midtown loft our hostess had rented, we hesitated. The building looked rundown and somewhat ominous in its isolation from the more heavily trafficked parts of the city. But we had come too far to turn back, so we climbed the wide, stone steps, took the elevator up to the fifth floor, and paid forty dollars to walk through an entryway strewn with shiny, metallic streamers.

Inexperienced as we were in the sex party social scene, we were among the first to arrive, and we huddled against each other in a corner of the main room as our hostess finished setting out bowls of Twizzlers and pretzels. The only other guest at that point was an older man wearing ass-less leather chaps and a matching leather cowboy hat, seated astride a bar stool on the far side of the room. I relinquished my bottle of wine to a girl with multicolored hair standing behind a small bar, ready with an assortment of markers so she could label guests' liquor bottles. I was relieved when more people finally began to arrive.

Some were dressed much like me: simply, in jeans and low-cut tops. Others had corsets and waist cinchers and bustiers, lacy, elaborately boned, and paired with fishnets and heels. Other outfits were even more extravagantly crafted. We wandered around the loft trying not to gawk.

Unsure about what to do with ourselves, we explored the space, pushing through beaded doorways to find rooms set aside for a wide variety of kinks. We found an S&M room, which would later be used for flogging, bondage, and humiliation. For those at the more playful end of the sexual spectrum, a tickle room stood as a paean to everything light and fluffy. Feathers were strung on streamers and hung from the ceiling, while smooshy cocoons were stacked in corners. There was also a room containing one enormous bed. It was intended for group sex but was first being used for a hands-on oral sex seminar called Sword Swallowing 101.

We had come for a sex party, but—aside from some of the more unconventional attire—the whole thing seemed like your typical cocktail party . . . at first. We settled into a deep, velvet sofa to chat with another couple while someone working the event came around offering absinthe. I stuck to my wine, sucking it down from a clear, plastic cup. The Pinot Grigio burned sweet and acidic down the back of my throat, landing in my gut and spreading a warmth that settled into all of my limbs, imparting the blessed relief of alcohol-enabled self-assurance.

As people eased deeper into the evening, the first signs that this was not your average cocktail party began to emerge. A man with slicked-back, black hair, wearing a gleaming leather skirt and a corset, held a woman's bare foot aloft in one hand, caressed it, kissed each toe tip and let his mouth travel along its arch all the way up to the ankle. On another couch, a curvaceous woman in black, lacy lingerie was on all fours; she shimmied her shoulders as her partner smacked her backside to the rhythm of the techno music. Nearby, another man casually draped his arm around a girl's shoulders and cupped her breasts, which were overflowing the tight confines of her bustier.

I was the type of person who felt uncomfortable kissing in public, or even holding hands. But I wasn't appalled by what was going on around me. Rather, looking around, I wished I could be as unselfconscious as the other guests, led by desire rather than feeling restrained by the noise in my head. But ever since Travis, I couldn't help but hear a litany of put-downs and disparagements in my head every time I took off my clothes. For the most part, I was too distracted by this interior cataloguing of my faults to be fully open to any all-consuming rushes of desire. How could these people put their appetites on display like this, in front of so many people? How could they feel so free when I couldn't even let go with just the two of us in a room together?

I ventured to the snack table alone, ending up in conversation with the only person there who was dressed like a CPA. In his khakis and button-down shirt, he was another sex party noob, and he seemed even more spellbound by the scene around us than I was. We watched together as a statuesque woman wearing nothing but a thong lay herself down on a table in the center of the room, ice cream cones on each bare breast. Seized with sudden courage, my new acquaintance leapt forward to sample the wares, resurfacing with smears of vanilla and chocolate all over his nose and mouth.

I eventually made my way back to Michael, where he was chatting with the couple who seemed to think nothing of public breast-fondling. Emboldened by this, Michael looked at me as he stretched an arm across my shoulders, his hand inching toward my cleavage. I looked at him sternly and, chastened, he clasped his hands in his lap.

But after a while, the atmosphere created by the abundance of bare flesh and the playful eroticism on display throughout the room crept up on me. I could feel my pudenda, slick and swollen, pressing against the crotch of my jeans, pulsing against the denim as I shifted in my chair. It had been so long since I'd felt this way.

Michael sensed a shift in the wind, and we excused ourselves from our conversation in order to find a dark corner. And then there, through one doorway, in a dark, empty room that was more like a liminal space between play areas, we clutched at each other, collapsing onto a brown, leather couch, pulling at each other's waistbands, grasping at body parts.

As we thrust and rubbed against each other, our desire nearly blinding us to our surroundings, I noticed that someone had appeared in the doorway. This person seemed surprised to find anyone else in that dark room, but also pleased, and he made himself comfortable, leaning against the door jamb to watch, sharing a smile with me when he caught my eye.

Though once upon a time, I had pushed Michael away when he'd kissed me in the middle of a dance club, though there had once been a time when I would automatically pull my hand away from his as we walked down the street, I turned back to Michael and I kept going. After turning away from him for so long, to turn toward him in that moment was a release in itself. Later, enlivened by that feeling of sexual abandon, I threw myself back into sex writing, trying to chase that feeling, grasp it, hold onto it forever.

We went to a handful of sex parties after that first one, never again experiencing what we experienced before. After swinging by an erotic art opening at a small downtown gallery one night, we went to a porn release party at the Pussycat Lounge, where we watched burlesque performers bump and grind to Esthero and dodged the free porn DVDs that were tossed out to the crowd. I went to a lingerie launch party and convinced Michael to buy me the set I most lusted over. I wore it once. We went to a cuddle party another night and learned that cuddle parties made us both extremely uncomfortable. That form of closeness and intimacy was something we'd always been able to give each other, and it seemed odd to seek it out in a group of strangers. After an awkward exchange in which I sat astride another attendee, massaging his shoulders as he and my husband talked about web development, I had to admit to myself that I was out of my element.

We snuck out near the end when everyone piled up into one large mass at the center of the room for the closing "cuddle puddle."

Michael acquiesced to all of this, and not because he was necessarily interested in New York's sex-positive scene. He would have been perfectly happy to stay in at night, engaging in the most vanilla of sex acts, just me, him, and maybe my vibrator. But he knew I was searching for something, and he knew it would only benefit our intimate relationship if I found it. And so, he did even the things that made him uncomfortable.

One of those things was the *Women's Health* photo shoot. A sexuality educator I met at our first sex party (the Sword Swallowing 101 instructor) was writing an article in which she was to assign "sex homework" to couples who were struggling with their sex lives. As I was always struggling, I volunteered. I thought: *maybe she can fix me*. We were then tasked with going to a sex shop together and testing out a toy we had never tried. The logic was that the ecstasy I experienced on my own with a clitoral vibrator might be successfully incorporated into partner play, leading to my own sexual fulfillment during intercourse. So we took a field trip to Babeland's Soho location, picked up under-the-bed restraints and a vibrating cock ring, and gave both their due diligence. Which was fine. It was no cure, but it wasn't necessarily unpleasant.

The assignment, however, did not end there. After we finished our homework, we had to coordinate a photo shoot in the city with the magazine's photographers where they had us posing awkwardly with whips and ticklers. And therein lay the problem. Because one day, while at work, one of Michael's coworkers spotted him in her latest issue of *Women's Health* and, soon, the entire office knew. Michael became, temporarily, the butt of many jokes involving buzzing sounds and double entendres. His more conservative coworkers were flat-out offended.

"I felt awkward," Michael told me years later, when I asked him about the experience for a blog post. "But I was still proud of you. Some people poked fun for a couple days, but most people were probably jealous."

So I continued to review a variety of sex toys and sexy how-tos, trying out vibrators that heated up, trying out vibrators that buzzed in time to the music playing on my iPod, even trying out the since-discontinued Sexerciseball. This last one was the most challenging for me, as I did not enjoy using sex toys for penetration. By this point, I was already grappling with the afore-mentioned sharp, shooting pain during intercourse, but I hoped that pushing myself in this way might eliminate the pain I had come to suspect was fear-induced.

I decided to take a different approach. While interning at an online magazine that specialized in content about sex, I received a press release from an artist who drew intimate portraits. *Maybe all of my problems in the bedroom stem from body image issues,* I thought to myself, remembering the many ways in which Travis had cut me down during our brief but intense relation-ship. I pitched my editors a personal essay in which I would explore these issues by posing nude. They gave me the go-ahead, and soon I found myself on the door-step of the artist who happened to live the next town over from me. I arrived dressed in my approximation of sexy—a charcoal gray pencil skirt and calf-high black leather boots—over-prepared as always, carrying a bag filled with an assortment of blankets, pajama combinations, and lingerie.

He led me up to his attic studio and I lay my coat and my large duffel bag off to the side as he explained his process to me, speaking of the initial quick sketches we would do before settling on a final pose. We discussed the length of time it would take for him to complete the final product, as well as the benefits of some positions versus others based upon how exhausting or uncomfortable it can be to remain still for an extended period of time, limbs shaking, growing numb.

After talking logistics, he suggested we begin. I was shy at the prospect of disrobing in front of a complete stranger, so I started slowly, pulling my sweater up and over my head. My hot pink bra screamed against the pale cream of my skin as I stared at a paint spot on the loose floorboards, avoiding his eyes. I couldn't stop thinking about my curves, my muffin top, the way my thighs rubbed together.

After striking several poses, I unzipped my boots and pulled them off, and then carefully slipped my tights down to my ankles. Stepping out of them, I rolled them up, and placed them neatly to the side. I started to inch down the zipper on my skirt, considered removing it, but then I paused, not ready for the next step.

Instead, I raised my arms above my head and grabbed opposite elbows, drawing my shoulders back and thrusting my chest forward in an attempt to look flirty. I suspected that I looked ridiculous, but he never let on, allowing me to blunder my way through a series of increasingly awkward poses. Finally, having exhausted the full repertoire of postures—or at least some facsimile thereof—that I had maybe seen while bingeing *America's Next Top Model*, I tugged on my fleece Cookie Monster pajama pants before taking off my skirt, careful not to flash a single inch of bare skin. As if to make up for this, I unclasped my bra, pushed the straps off my shoulders, and tossed it to the side. Heat crept up my neck, my cheeks, even as my nipples hardened in the cool air. My breasts were firm, aware of every draft, every movement.

After some time, I pushed down my pajama pants. I dropped my cotton briefs to the floor. Then I pulled a blanket off the couch and wrapped it around my body, drawing it tight around my shoulders, taking a moment to gather myself. I walked over to a pallet on the floor covered in sheets and pillows and even more blankets, and lay down on my stomach, propped up on my elbows. I watched him as he leaned over his paper, pencil scrabbling across the page. At the two-minute mark, he looked up and nodded at me. After a moment of hesitation, I shifted onto my back. I let the blanket slip lower.

I held my breath. I thought of Travis. I thought of him ridiculing me, mocking my full patch of pubic hair. I held my breath some more. I considered covering up.

Instead, my legs opened several inches, and I found I could feel the heat radiating from the nearby space heater on my clitoris. Newly mindful of various sensations in my body, my anxious mind began to quiet. The room was silent, save for the whir of the space heaters, and the soft whisper of the artist turning the pages of his notepad, running his pencils across the paper.

Eventually, we sat beside each other on the floor, and he fanned his sketches out in front of me. I didn't recognize myself in the drawings. They revealed a version of me I had never been able to see. But we picked the one we liked the most and, for the rest of the day, he painted as I lay stretched out on the floor. By the end of our time together, I barely even noticed I was naked.

The artist came to our condo when the painting was complete and, when he unveiled it to the both of us, I could tell Michael was impressed. There were my soft, pendulous breasts. One pink nipple winking out from behind the edge of a blanket. The cleft where my thighs met my vulva. It was a reminder, for Michael, of everything lying in wait beneath my clothes, and seeing it made him want me. But what I loved was how beautiful I looked, how relaxed and unconstrained. For so long, Travis's every slight had been at the back of my mind, a slow poison that burned my gut and made me tense up every time I looked in the mirror or saw a photograph of myself, every time Michael pulled down my jeans, peeled off my underpants, unclasped my bra, bent to the space between my legs. But the woman in this painting did not hate her body, nor was her self-worth wrapped up in the gaze of others. Looking at this watercolor version of me I could almost return to how I felt in the artist's studio as the day had darkened into evening— serene and self-assured in the body I'd been given.

Unfortunately, the effects of my intimate portrait weren't permanent. Every time I caught sight of the me I still hated—in the bathroom mirror, in bed—the painting of me seemed more like a lie: a visual representation of my wishful thinking.

Over time, I began to think that immersive sex writing might not be enough. What made things even more difficult was the fact that I was not necessarily trying to reclaim something I had lost. Rather, I was chasing something I never really had. Something I felt I *should* have. Was success even possible? Was a fulfilling sex life possible? Was a healthy intimate relationship, whatever that might mean, even possible?

But I continued the chase. I let "sex writer" become the thing that defined me. I kept throwing myself into new experiences in the hopes that things would click into place, that I would be brought back to that magical state of wanting I'd experienced at my very first sex party.

I also entertained the possibility that this might be about more than just my first, shitty sexual experience. More than just a byproduct of the mental wall I had erected to protect myself from the things that had already happened, the things that might happen again. I considered the fact that there might be something physically wrong with me. I cast a wider net as I continued to look for answers.

In addition to writing sex toy reviews and attending erotic events, I saw Dr. Jill every week. I always left her office feeling lighter but, when it came to sex, nothing she said led to the type of revelation that I needed. I tried homeopathy and hypnotherapy. But the remedy the homeopath gave me had no discernible effect on my libido *or* my pain. And I couldn't bring myself to continue paying for hypnotherapy sessions that felt like nothing more than light naps.

One day, I told my gynecologist about the pain I'd

been experiencing. At my annual pap smear appointment, I admitted to her that I felt pain during intercourse. I asked her if there was something wrong with me down there. If there was something she could do, something that could be fixed.

She slid the speculum out of me. A paper robe barely covered me, the bottoms of my feet were cold, and gooseflesh pimpled up on my legs. She crouched back over me, shined a penlight into the cavern between my legs, swung the tiny light back and forth. She stuck a finger into my vagina to feel around inside, hmmm'd under her breath and, after what felt like a cursory amount of time, straightened up and moved over to the sink to peel off her gloves and wash her hands.

"Everything seems fine to me," she said. She wiped her hands with a paper towel. "But if you'd like to pursue this, you could always get a transabdominal ultrasound."

She scribbled something onto her prescription pad, ripped off the sheet, and handed it to me. I slipped it into my purse, feeling renewed hope despite her dismissive demeanor.

Several weeks later, I sat in the waiting room at the ultrasound facility, my legs pressed together, my Kegels clenched. I had been required to drink twenty-four ounces of water at least an hour before my appointment, and they were running late. When I was finally led to an examining room, I worried that every movement I made might make me pee my pants. They spread gel across my abdomen and ran the transducer over the bulge of my belly, pressing gently to get a clearer picture, and I clenched my thighs together desperately.

When it was finally over, I had the most glorious pee of my life, and then the ultrasound technician presented her findings.

Everything looks completely normal, she said.

I saw nothing out of the ordinary, she said.

Maybe your pain is psychological, she said.

It was several more years before the pain went away, and this miraculous breakthrough had nothing to do with my sex writing. In fact, my sex writing became much less personal over that span of time, much less immersive and experimental, as I shifted focus to help sexuality professionals translate their research for a wider, less academic audience.

During this time, Michael and I began trying to build a family. Because of this, we upped our sexual frequency to coincide with my periods of ovulation, having sex at least once a week and on the weeks when I was ovulating doing it every other day.

We didn't do it for pleasure. It was sex with a *purpose*.

But something happened to me during that time.

No, having sex more frequently did not light a fire under my guttering libido. But it did make me used to it, used to the regular, recurrent penetration. It did help me relax into it. And as my mind relaxed, I stopped tensing up my pelvic muscles. And as my muscles relaxed, I stopped experiencing pain. Stopped anticipating it. Simple as that.

Or perhaps not so simple when you consider how long it took for me to get to that point. Years later, I would learn that sexual pain in itself is not so simple.

Years after I stopped hurting, I would come to interview leading researchers in the areas of genital, vulvar,
and pelvic floor pain, and I would come to learn that
such pain was a biopsychosocial issue,[3] attributable to
biological factors, psychological factors, social factors,
or some combination thereof.[4] I would learn that the
complexity of this pain—in addition to existing gender
biases in medical diagnosing—make identifying and
treating it exceptionally difficult. Those who have a
strong understanding of sexual pain now know that
managing it requires a multi-pronged approach, one
that can include talk therapy, mindfulness exercises,
physical therapy, and any number of other methods.

At the time when my own pain finally ceased, I had
already engaged in hours of talk therapy. My yoga and
meditation practice had certainly taught me mindfulness. But clearly, up until then, a piece of the puzzle had
still been missing. Despite all of my magical thinking,
and all of my flailing about from specialist to specialist,
I was only destined to stumble upon it accidentally,
when it was furthest from my mind.

In the end, all it took to fix this part of me was a
mental sleight of hand, a radical shift in focus from

3   Talli Y Rosenbaum, MSc, Ellen Barnard, MSSW, and Myrtle
    Wilhite, MD, MS. "Psychosexual Aspects of Vulvar Disease."
    Clinical Obstetrics and Gynecology 58, no. 3 (2015): 551–55.
    doi:10.1097/grf.0000000000000136.

4   Jacob Bornstein, MD, MPA, Andrew T. Goldstein, MD, Colleen
    K. Stockdale, MD, MS, Sophie Bergeron, PhD, Caroline Pukall,
    PhD, Denniz Zolnoun, MD, MPH, and Deborah Coady, MD
    "2015 ISSVD, ISSWSH and IPPS Consensus Terminology
    and Classification of Persistent Vulvar Pain and Vulvodynia."
    Obstetrics & Gynecology 127, no. 4 (2016): 745–51. doi:10.1097
    /aog.0000000000001359.

wanting to enjoy sex to wanting to have a baby. Baby-making sex. Who would have thought that the most dispassionate, high-stakes lovemaking of my life would be exactly the form of physical therapy I needed most?

6 | MY MOST COMPLICATED RELATIONSHIP IS WITH MY BODY

"Are you pregnant?" the owner of the dry cleaner asked me as I slid my clothes across the counter and waited for her to draw up my receipt. She beamed at me, excited for my future. "When are you due?"

I smiled back at her, trying not to look as appalled as I felt. "Nope," I told her. "Not pregnant." I wrapped my arms around my body. Looked down at the counter.

Which is when she should have dropped it. But then: "Are you sure?"

"Pretty sure," I said, because I didn't know what else to say.

She made a *hmmm* sound, like maybe I didn't know my body as well as I thought I did, and then she handed me my slip of paper.

My face was hot when I turned to go. I pushed my way out the door, the bells that hung from the doorknob jingling. I tugged at my empire-waist tunic top as I walked briskly to my car, worrying that it looked too much like a maternity top. *So much for my clothes,* I thought to myself, trying to make peace with the fact that I would never see them again. *I can never go back there.*

I have never been one of those long and lithe women who wear a size zero and make maxi skirts look like high fashion. But once upon a time, I was a perfectly adequate size eight, and it wasn't such a leap of faith to let my legs grow long and bare out of a pair of shorts, or to wear a bikini in public. Even when I went to college, I only expanded marginally to a size ten. I often wandered around my apartment in a pair of plaid boxer shorts. I went to parties without a bra.

But then I met Michael. Much of our courtship took place at McDonalds, where I ate Big Macs and fries, the sauce from my burger ever collecting at the corner of my mouth until I licked it clean. Sometimes, I had one or two of his McNuggets. Afterward, we would return to his house and watch our beloved B-horror movies in bed, my body heavy in the aftermath of our fast food binge. As I lay in his bed, watching *Dead Alive* or *Evil Dead 2*, I swear I could feel my waistline expanding.

Some time later, after we got engaged and bought a one-bedroom condo together, we had an argument about the division of labor in our relationship. "Nothing you make even tastes good!" he shouted as I listed out all of the housework I was in charge of, including dinner. I was driving my car down the highway at the time and, furious, I considered pulling over to the shoulder, forcing him to get out and walk. Instead, I simply stopped cooking for a year.

We spent that time subsisting on pasta and pizza and takeout lo mein. Soon enough, I was thirty pounds heavier than I wanted to be. The waistband of my jeans dug into the flesh at my hips, and my breasts overflowed the cups of my bras and slopped out underneath the band that I pulled tight around my torso. My pants went up a size. And then they went up again. A trip to the mall could render me tearful in a claustrophobic fitting room, my lungs constricted, my skin hot and prickly. I hated the body I saw in the mirror. I hated myself for allowing my weight gain to get so far.

By the time I started cooking again, making an effort to eat healthfully (or at least healthi*er*), it was too late. I wasn't gaining anymore, but I didn't lose weight either.

The expansion of my belly, my waist, and my torso coincided with all of the other ways in which I was learning to loathe my body. For one thing, the small blips of desire I had been experiencing every so often disappeared entirely. I would much rather sit propped up in bed, a book resting in the crease between my ribs and my stomach, than peel off my pajama pants and my cotton bikini briefs and pull my husband close. I didn't seem to *need* that intimate human contact anymore— didn't feel that natural human drive for it. After all, if I ever felt that electric zip pulsing through my vulva, the zip that only an orgasm could cure, a quick session with my Jimmyjane smoothie vibrator, its shaft pressed insistently against my clitoral hood, could do the job better than Michael. If I ever paused to consider what this meant about the state of my marriage, I ended up twisted in a cycle of guilt and frustration that only dampened my libido more.

My body ceased showing signs of physical arousal as well. Where once, long ago, I might have occasion-ally grown slick and tingling and achy from the brush of skin against skin, my vulva was now a dry, barren wasteland. I required huge glops of personal lubricant during sex. Its oily excess settled into the valleys between my fingers and left palm prints on his shoulder blades, on my thighs.

And then there was everything that came after that. The bottles of Lexapro and Xanax I tossed into the trash alongside my birth control pills when we finally decided to start a family. The three and a half years of infertility that followed. The depression that crept back in without the medication to keep it at bay, long expanses of hopelessness, frequent flare-ups of anger, periods during which I was completely without affect, when I didn't even know what I was working toward anymore.

At this time, it almost didn't matter that I couldn't see myself as a sexual being. It didn't matter that I hated the person I saw in the mirror, all bulges and broadness and ill-fitting clothing. I couldn't see the point in trying to acquire a healthy sense of sexuality, a healthy body. The one thing I had always wanted—to be a mother—was out of my reach. This seemed to me to be my body's final betrayal.

The slim stitches that held my marriage together began to pull loose, fall out. In bed at night, I piled blankets on top of me. My skin was cold as we curled away from each other in the dark, our backbones six inches apart.

During this shaky part of my marriage, I found yoga. Which sounds like a yuppie cliché in the style of *Eat, Pray, Love*, but it truly saved me.

I had taken a few classes in the past, at the gym. I

stumbled my way through pose after pose, a few beats behind everyone else, as the people around me held plank without breaking a sweat and effortlessly tipped over into crow pose, an arm balance that still eludes me.

I spent a year following yoga DVDs in the living room of our small condominium, my movements bearing only a slight resemblance to what was happening on the screen. One time, while doing a DVD from yoga star Shiva Rea, I watched her lay down on her back and lift her legs up and over her head into plow pose. Her hips just kept on hinging, unimpeded by such obstacles as belly fat or love handles or sagging breasts, and her toes eventually came to kiss the floor behind her head. When she reached the full extension of the pose, she looked like a perfectly folded piece of origami, ends carefully creased tight.

When I tried to do the same pose, the waistband of my pajama pants cut uncomfortably into the area between my belly button and pubic bone. The fabric pulled taut at my thighs. My toes hovered in the air, several feet above the floor. My muffin top and my breasts heaved themselves in the direction of my face. I struggled to breathe.

As I strained to reach the floor behind me, Shiva Rea moved smoothly into knee-to-ear pose, a pose that took her folded-flat origami body and crumpled it up into a tiny ball. To do this, she wrapped her arms around the backs of her thighs and then simply bent her legs, letting her knees rest on the floor on either side of her head. "Yeah right," I gasped, mere moments away from toppling over. It felt as if all of my organs were being squeezed tight in someone's fist.

Michael walked in from the dining room and stood behind me, squinting at the TV screen and then looking down at me. I could see, out of the corner of my eye, his legs swimming in skinny jeans that were too big on him, the hard points of his hips visible through his shirt. I heard him lift a glass to his lips and take a long, slow sip.

"She's doing it better than you," he finally said before continuing on to the kitchen. I tried not to hate him.

It was later, during the time when we were digging into the guts of our relationship, that I first went to a yoga studio. I was progressing decently on my own, but I wanted someone to stamp out any bad habits I might be unconsciously developing, to fix my alignment, and to push me harder than I pushed myself.

I found a studio just five minutes away from our condo that offered five-dollar community classes on Friday nights, taught by yoga teacher trainees. I immediately liked the laid-back atmosphere of the studio. While in the past I had been intimidated by the fitness enthusiasts at the gym, the people at the studio were more relaxed. More forgiving. The teachers stressed the importance of listening to your body and doing what served it best. Class attendees, meanwhile, were having fun. They weren't there to get six-pack abs or drop down several pants sizes. They were more focused on learning something new. Learning what their bodies were capable of.

I started paying full price for the classes taught by the certified instructors, going multiple times a week to try out various teaching styles. When one teacher got me up into headstand only a few classes in, I was hooked. Feeling my legs float up overhead, my arms and abs trembling with the hard work, was exhilarating. I immediately purchased an unlimited class package and began attending class four to six times a week.

Looking back, it's obvious I was running away from my difficulties at home. With problem piled upon problem, I couldn't help but feel sorry for myself. Where before I had spurned my body, seeing it as the source of so much anguish, now I turned inward, working everything out through sweat and breath and muscle. My home was a landmine. My yoga mat was shelter.

As I spent more time delving into my yoga practice, I could feel myself growing stronger, more flexible. More sane. I may have inherited my mother's thunder thighs, but my legs were strong enough to pull off a mean crescent lunge. I may have felt wide, bulky, and ungainly, but none of that bulk got in the way when I opened my hips and folded into pigeon pose. I may not have considered myself to be someone with endurance but, only a few months into my time at the studio, I pushed and sweated my way through a twelve-hour yogathon.

And even after all of this—*because* of all of this—I wanted more. While Michael seemed to have no problem looking at me and seeing someone fuckable, even in the thick of our marital problems, I still wasn't satisfied with what I saw. I still wasn't comfortable removing my clothes without first turning off the lights and sliding beneath the sheets, wriggling out of pants and tops like Houdini wriggling out of a straitjacket while wrapped up in chains and locked in a box. Yoga was getting me closer to a place where I might prance around my room wearing only bikini briefs, but it was still a work in progress. It felt good to continue doing that work.

Beyond that, focusing on my breath and on my practice helped me to forget all the ways in which we were *really* struggling at home. I wanted to go deeper into my practice, so deep that all I'd see were my mat and my toes, all I'd hear were my inhales and exhales. The teacher who got me up into my first headstand had been saying for months that I would eventually become a teacher. Like it was an inevitability. Like it was fate. About two years into my time at the studio, I entered the owner's teacher training program. I had no intention of teaching—the thought of leading a group of people in *anything* terrified me—but I was counting on the immersive nature of the program to make my practice even stronger.

On the first day of yoga teacher training, we slipped into the studio for the 9 a.m. class, rolling out our mats alongside the regular practitioners. I placed two blocks at the front of my mat, then folded up a blanket and sat on the edge of it, pelvis tilted forward, spine long. Resting my hands on my knees, I grew taller, inhaling long and slow through my nose, willing my body to relax more on every exhale. But I could feel the nervous energy coursing through my stomach, my chest, my fingertips. I had been coming to this 9 a.m. advanced class taught by the studio owner for a year, but this morning marked the start of something different.

She took us through an initial centering, making her way through her dharma talk, guiding us through the lengthening of our breath. We set our intentions. We *om'd*. Then we rolled forward onto all fours and immediately pressed up into downward dog, bicycling out our legs, broadening our upper backs, pressing forward through our knuckles. We spent the next hour and a half pushing our way through *vinyasas*, sun salutations, and a mix of forward folds and back bends. With five minutes to spare, we splayed ourselves open into spinal twists, lingering on each side before finally sprawling out into *savasana*. After the final *om,* the students around us rolled up their mats and poured out of the studio. My fellow teacher trainees and I had seven hours left to go.

We spent that day learning the basics: how to put together a dharma talk, how to lead a class in *om,* how to teach a variety of breathing exercises. We drew up flash cards of the most common yoga poses, writing down the names in English on one side and in Sanskrit on the other. We started to learn how to adjust our students in certain poses in order to improve their alignment, or just to make them feel good. We started teaching each other round robin style, each of us taking the lead for five minutes before moving on to the next person. When we were finally dismissed at the end of the day, we were all punch drunk.

The next five months progressed much like this. We practiced yoga for hours, and then we practiced teaching. We pressed down on each other's hips in child's pose and pulled spines longer in downward dog. We spent hours watching anatomy videos, and even had an anatomy expert come in and talk to us several times. We learned meditation techniques and we read and analyzed ancient Buddhist texts.

As the weeks passed, my body changed. My legs

grew leaner and my calves more muscular. My biceps and the muscles beneath the pooch of my stomach grew harder. My hamstrings loosened, and my heels touched the ground in downward dog for the first time since I started practicing yoga. Though I would likely hyperventilate if you asked me to go for a run or climb multiple flights of stairs, I felt like a warrior. The things my body was capable of astounded me. I felt proud of it. I felt at peace with its curves.

I felt at peace, period. Or at least better equipped to manage my interior roller coaster of emotions. Learning how to build a pose from the ground up—how to move my muscles into their proper alignment using tiny adjustments—gave me patience and a greater awareness of my body and its inner workings. I got to a place where I could relax certain parts of my body just by thinking it. Learning to focus on the breath and the body also gave me an inner quiet. A new ability to respond to things without immediate, unthinking, emotion-driven reaction.

These newfound skills would come to serve me in the bedroom, and not just because of some acquired nudge-nudge-wink-wink flexibility. Rather, my practice enabled me to relax my pelvic floor muscles, something that contributed heavily to the eradication of my sexual pain. Plus, I became able to notice things—to increase my focus and exclude all of the normal background noise of life. I became able to notice and acknowledge how good it felt when Michael ran his palms down my back or pressed his pelvis insistently into mine, stimulating my clitoris without direct contact. I was able to stay with those feelings without getting distracted by the cats at the foot of the bed or the laundry on the floor or the emails that still needed to be sent. Sex could actually be pleasurable.

Still it took me a long time to realize the sexual benefits I was receiving from my practice. I remained distracted by the difficulties in my marriage. And by the fact that, even as my body finally seemed to be moving past the physical and psychological reverberations of my relationship with Travis, it was finding other ways to thwart me. As I made my way through teacher training, I was concurrently going through fertility treatments. By the time I earned my teaching certification, we had tried intrauterine insemination (IUI) twice, and had failed both times. I couldn't fathom what was wrong. The ultrasound technician told me that my ovaries looked beautiful.

Michael eventually got a recommendation for a different urologist and we learned that my body wasn't the problem. I understood that this was a blow to his masculinity but, at the same time, it felt good to know that my body was operating correctly. That in this one way, at least, I wasn't defective.

It would be at least half a year before we could try artificial insemination again. We took advantage of the break in the infertility treatment process to take a two-week trip to Greece and Italy. Our time there made me grateful for my yoga practice and the ways in which it had reshaped my body and made me stronger.

When we arrived in Santorini after a few days in Karpathos for an old friend's traditional Greek wedding, we found our luggage hadn't made the trip. After filing paperwork at the airport, we took a shuttle to our cliff-side hotel. The sun beat down, bright and relentless, and I stared at the other hotel guests as they glided about the pool.

We decided to hike the path up the cliff face to see if we could find provisions at the nearest small village. I had on jeans, socks, and sneakers. I was wearing the only pair of underpants that hadn't been packed away in my luggage. My feet boiled in my walking sneakers, growing slick and slimy. My legs strained. My lungs contracted like a wheezing bellow.

When we finally reached the village, we were able to find toothbrushes, toothpaste, razors, and other essentials. I got a cheap pair of flip-flops. Michael chose from a selection of swim trunks, and also grabbed a tote bag and two beach blankets. But the only bathing suit I was able to find was a string bikini, packed up in crinkly plastic so I couldn't even try it on.

Never in my life had I worn a string bikini, even when I was at my skinniest.

I bought it anyway.

We made our way back down the path, the soles of our shoes sliding along the pebbles in the dirt as our calves strained against the steep decline.

Back at the hotel, I peeled off my clothes, the sweat in the folds of my vulva sticking to the cotton bikini briefs that had been on my body for two days. I used the cheap razor I'd purchased to clean up my bikini line. I pulled on the bikini.

"How does it look?" I asked Michael, looking at the entire length of me in the mirror, trying to determine what would win out: my muffin top or my need for a cool dip in the pool.

"I think you look great," he said, because he values his life. I tilted my head at my reflection, wishing the bikini bottoms weren't so low cut, wondering what the chances were that I'd flash my butt crack.

"I guess it's not as bad as I thought," I said. "It doesn't fit perfectly, but . . . I looked at all of the places where my body had hardened, the muscles growing taut and tough. "I haven't worn a bikini in years. But this is making me think I could actually pull one off. Not this one maybe, but . . ."

We left our room, making our way to the pool. The feel of the water slipping across my skin as I slid in was glorious. I switched back to my one-piece when our luggage caught up with us late the next day, but what I'd seen in the mirror the day before planted yet another seed of confidence in my body.

I spent the rest of the trip especially conscious of my physicality. Yoga had given me a greater sense of body awareness, but I never had the opportunity to test my strength outside of the studio. On this trip, we climbed the cliff path many times to catch the bus into the more lively sections of Santorini. We spent a day on a pirate ship, which took us to a dormant volcano, the most arduous hike I'd ever undertaken. Afterward, we sailed to a hot spring, diving off the side of the boat into the bathwater-warm sea. And when we were done in Santorini, we flew to Italy, where we spent days walking the streets of Florence, the dust from the cobblestones turning our feet black. By the time we returned to New Jersey, I was spent.

Two months later, I was pregnant. I had been teaching yoga for five months by that point, despite my initial stated objective to focus on my own practice. I substitute-taught at four different gyms and had my own classes at three different studios. I also taught a group of women at a country club in Short Hills. I squeezed in my own practice when I could. When I learned I was pregnant, I had no intention of slowing down. Yoga had been good to me and I wanted to continue sharing it with others. I also hoped that the flexibility and body awareness and breathing techniques I was cultivating in my own practice would help the labor go more smoothly.

At the same time, I was constantly terrified I would somehow damage the fetus. And I received a lot of conflicting advice from my various teachers.

"No twists, obviously," said Brian, my Monday morning teacher. "And nothing on the belly. And no jumping either," he said, referring to jump-ups and jump-backs, and also to the way in which I cartwheeled up into my handstands. He was always concerned that I might be doing something dangerous.

"You already have a strong practice," said my other teacher, who had continued teaching and practicing and popping up into inversions until the day she popped out her own baby. "You can do anything you were doing before, up until it doesn't feel good anymore." She showed me how to modify certain poses as my stomach grew bigger, and how to use a collection of props to get the best possible *savasana*. She helped me maintain my regular practice for as long as possible.

"The first thing to go will be legs up the wall," she said knowingly, referring to an inversion where we lay flat on our backs, butts up against the seam between floor and wall, legs reaching toward the ceiling. Pregnant women tend to feel discomfort if they lie flat on their backs. But I never lost legs up the wall. And I gained the understanding that there are no hard and fast rules, and that every woman experiences pregnancy differently.

I did eventually stop going to regular classes, midway through my third trimester. I reached a point where, as I struggled to step back into lunges or sink into chair pose, I just felt uncomfortable. My belly was, unsurprisingly, often in the way. And if I drew in my belly too tightly while rising up to stand, a cramp would sizzle across my abdomen. My energy was also near empty. With all these changes to my body, my practice was no longer serving me. So even though my teacher told me prenatal yoga would bore me, I started attending a weekly class at my OB/GYN's office. It wasn't the same, but it was something.

I did keep teaching, though, continuing to demonstrate poses as best I could. One time, while piking down from a headstand, a fellow teacher marveled that she could still see my abs, even though I was pregnant. "She's pregnant!?" another student exclaimed, and I couldn't help but smile at her disbelief. It didn't seem that long since my dry cleaner had mistaken my soft and pillowy curves for a sign of pregnancy. At my country club class, demonstrating several ways in which to get up into headstand, a student commented that my baby was going to come out an acrobat. These remarks brought me a sense of satisfaction. My belly was expanding, my ankles turning to cankles, my breasts leaping up a cup size, yet I had never loved my body more.

It didn't hurt that my pregnancy was easy. Though

I felt a low-level nausea 24/7 well into the second trimester, I never vomited. And there were no medical complications. It wasn't until the latter half of my third trimester that I started looking with desperation toward the day I might go into labor. And only because I had reached the point where I could no longer get comfortable in bed.

When I did go into labor, it was the middle of the night, the pain so excruciating that I vomited. I threw up three more times at the hospital before they wheeled me into the room where I would give birth. I moaned and clenched my body with every contraction, and Michael moved to the side of my bed and held my hand. "Squeeze as hard as you need to," he said. Instead, I kicked my legs, pressing the soles of my feet into the metal bars at the foot of the bed.

"Remember your breathing exercises," said my mom. I glared at her. My entire body arched off the bed as the pain arced through me. I prayed that I was close.

"You're at seven centimeters," said my doctor when she checked in on me some time later.

I looked at her in disbelief.

"No!" I shouted. "Give me the drugs," I gasped out.

Everything was easier after that, though they had to dial back the drugs when it came time to push. At the very end, it felt as if my daughter was stuck there at the opening of my vagina. That I would never be able to thrust her out. But then Emily burst forth in a wash of blood and vernix, and her warm, slippery body was placed against my bare chest. I held her there, my entire body stiff, afraid I might drop her. It seemed unbelievable that she was mine.

But she was. She was mine. A tiny human in her own right, finally separate from my body.

At the same time, though, she was still a part of me.

Emily took to breastfeeding immediately, her lips pulling at my nipple, her tiny fingers pressed against my collarbone. I had felt an ambivalence toward breast-feeding in the months leading up to her birth, trying to dodge all of the rhetoric that came from the "breast is best" evangelists. But I had still promised my husband I would try, so I did. It was a miracle to me, how Emily immediately found my nipple with her mouth, sucking for something that could sustain her. But I did not feel the maternal ecstasy so many had described. My nipples burned and bled and, that first night in the hospital, she vomited, expelling more blood than milk, black across the front of her onesie.

Over the course of the next few months, I swung back and forth between the glow of that forced inti-macy, the fact of her need, and an ache to have my body be my own again. She was cluster feeding then, falling asleep with my skin still in her mouth, and it hurt when I tried to pop my nipple out from between her lips.

At the very least, breastfeeding carried with it the added benefit of quicker post-pregnancy weight loss. When I was nursing Emily, I became even slimmer than I was before the pregnancy. But in seeing my body thin out again, I was eager to return to my yoga practice. I was trimmer, but I wanted to be hard again. Solid. Strong. I wanted to regain everything I lost in the midst of this postpartum mix of fragility, frailty, isolation, and exhaustion.

I was told, however, that I wasn't allowed to exercise for at least six weeks after the birth.

I furtively eased my way through gentle movement in our back room, a postnatal yoga DVD guiding me back to myself. Then, at my six-week checkup, my doctor hunched forward between my thighs, parting the lips of my vulva and gently feeling around inside me. She straightened up, pulling off her gloves and tossing them in the trash. "I think you should wait just a *few* more weeks," she said, making a note on her chart.

"To go to yoga!?" I asked, distressed.

"No, silly! To have sex!" she said, shaking her head and smiling.

I sank back into my chair, adjusted my robe, and sighed with relief. "Oh, thank god," I said. "That I can handle."

I picked my practice back up slowly. My first time back at the studio was like learning my body all over again. I moved cautiously. I wondered where my abs had gone. I gloried in the ability to just sit and breathe on the oasis that was my yoga mat. On the drive back home, I realized I had not thought about Emily for an entire hour. I immediately began missing her. It was my first time away from her since she had been born.

I also took Em to a Mommy and Me yoga class once a week. Mommy and Me was different. The movements were gentler. They felt good, but I was never able to successfully enjoy a *savasana*. Em would start crying and I would have to feed her or change her or rock her in my arms, my feet doing a two-step that became so much a part of my DNA that I moved through it even when I wasn't holding her.

But she loved it when I lay on my back, hugged my knees in to my chest, and balanced her on my shins, extending my legs out and drawing them back in, making her fly. At these times, her mouth gaped as wide as her face in silent, delirious laughter. Seeing her like that, I couldn't begrudge her my failure to find an instant of self-repose.

Back home, we fell into a rhythm of breastfeeding in which I managed to take her off each breast after fifteen minutes without stretching my nipple to within an inch of its life. Then I'd place her in her Rock n' Play and dance for her or let her nod off while I worked at my laptop. One day, four months in, she refused the breast. And she continued to refuse it for several days afterward. I felt panic, though I had presumably been counting down the days until I could stop nursing. It occurred to me that I enjoyed the closeness we shared during her feedings, that I had become used to being attached to her, that I had grown roots. I was relieved when, a few days later, she turned back toward me and fed from my breast. The hot weight of her in my arms made everything feel right again.

When she weaned herself for good about a month later, I felt more prepared. I continued pumping, freezing plastic baggies of my milk, lining them up in a Tupperware in the freezer. Eventually, I stopped that, too, letting the milk erupt in slim streams in the shower, sliding nipple guards into my bras until, one day, I didn't have to anymore.

With nursing at an end, the pounds slowly crept back on. My thighs pillowed out again and my stomach grew soft. With a child to care for, I couldn't get to the yoga studio as much as I used to, and I couldn't find the time to practice at home for more than fifteen minutes at a time. I strained to button my jeans over my belly button and I looked in the mirror, wondering when I would stop loving and hating and loving and hating and loving and hating my body. I wondered if I would ever be able to just be.

Though pregnancy and early motherhood marked the greatest transformation of my body I've ever undergone, my body is still changing. My ankles and the arches of my feet hurt when I get out of bed in the morning. Last year, I had to go to physical therapy twice a week for five weeks due to a recurrent, shooting pain beneath my kneecap attributed to deterioration of the cartilage. Then I turned my ankle, spraining it slightly. It still hurt months later, and the pain made some yoga poses impossible. I had to pull back from my yoga practice in general and, even a year later, I feel that my practice is not what it used to be. When I stop to think about all of this—these signs of aging though I am only thirty-seven—I feel as if I'm crumbling.

Some days I feel beautiful. Some days I feel ugly. Sometimes I look at myself and feel nothing. I just feel the knowledge that it is what it is.

I try not to express body hate in front of my daughter. I let her use my belly as a drum. I let her walk in on me in the bathroom. I teach her about her head and her toes and her thighs and her vulva, and I tell her that every part of her is stunning.

I am more accepting of my own body, too: how it looks, how it feels, how it performs. And I want her to feel that about herself, too. I want her to always feel that.

But maybe full acceptance isn't always possible. Maybe it's too hard. Maybe that's okay. Maybe this is the best one can hope for.

Not full acceptance, but a tentative peace.

7 | BETRAYED BY OUR BODIES

"You know we'll have to have sex, right?" my husband asked when we decided it was time to start a family. He was kidding, of course. Or halfway kidding. But it was a fair point. We were in the middle of another long dry spell. A few years into our marriage, entire months would often spin out without an iota of intimacy between us.

It was my fault. Of course it was my fault. I had been wrestling with my body for years, colliding up against its wants, its lacks, its limitations. I had felt betrayed by it over and over again, ever since the length of my legs and the curve of my ass had prompted Travis to take my virginity without first securing my permission.

At this point, between my increased weight and our mismatched libidos, I was no longer the woman my husband had married. On his behalf, I carried enough guilt and self-loathing for the both of us.

Still—and though our marriage was far from perfect—after three years of building a life together, we felt we were ready for the children we had both always wanted. So I let my birth control prescription lapse and got rid of the medication I had been taking for years in order to manage my chronic depression and anxiety. I ordered fertility-friendly lube in bulk from Amazon to combat my lack of physical arousal. I downloaded a free menstrual calendar application onto my phone and used it to track both my ovulation and the frequency with which we had sex. We scrambled to sell our one-bedroom condominium so we could afford to buy a house. We were both certain it wouldn't be long before we would need the extra space.

Condos were a tough sell back then. We had purchased ours at the height of the market, and its value had dropped exponentially in the years since, making it impossible to sell without incurring a huge loss. But it turned out not to matter. It seemed pregnancy wouldn't be as easy as we had expected either. For a year and a half, we tried, tracking my cycle on my phone, referring to times of ovulation as Sex Week, during which we would engage in perfunctory intercourse every other day. But every month, the telltale spotting appeared in my panties, physical proof that—once again—we weren't pregnant.

I started to feel hopeless, simply because it hurt less than having my hope crushed over and over and over again. And without my antidepressants, I drifted back toward a depression and irrational anger that lived beneath my skin, in my body. Back when I was searching for the right mix of antidepressants, before I gave them up entirely in the service of starting a family, I often experienced wild mood swings. Because of the unpredictability of my emotions, our relationship had always been somewhat volatile. I would swing between periods of affectless depression and whirlwinds of mania, with the periods of equanimity in between becoming shorter and shorter. It didn't take much for me to lose my temper and, in fact, it was my temper that motivated my parents to find me a therapist in the first place, during my adolescence. Now, faced with a problem I couldn't control, I felt anger at our circumstances. Anger at my body. I began pushing Michael away when he turned toward me in bed, running a hand down my arm, stealing a quick grope of my breast. I began picking fights with him.

My husband coped with his own disappointment at our continuing childlessness by avoiding me, to avoid my dark moods and my rage. He stayed out late every night, bar hopping with his coworkers and then stumbling into our dark condo at two or three in the morning. I lay in bed with my fingers clenching the coverlet, unable to sleep because of the fury and resentment and frustration that burned its way down my esophagus to land heavy and roiling in my stomach. Sometimes, I pretended to be asleep, fingernails digging into my palms, knuckles straining. But more often, I lashed out at him in the darkness, berating him for the distance he had created between us. "Not this again," he would say, pulling on his pajama pants, sliding into bed, and turning away from me. My hands would tremble. My gut would burn. I would stare at shadows on the ceiling and kick the sheets around instead of sleeping.

One time, while arguing with Michael in our cramped condo kitchen about his late nights and the thoughtlessness with which he'd been treating me, neglecting even to call and let me know he wouldn't be home until late, I inadvertently burned a batch of cookie bars that had been baking in the oven. As I hacked at the bars with a spatula, trying unsuccessfully to remove them from the pan, the heat in my body rising with frustration and fury, Michael said something that set me off and I just snapped. I flung his just-cleaned laundry onto the kitchen floor, dumped the cookie bars on top of his button-down shirts and dryer-warmed jeans, and stomped up and down on top of the whole mess, grinding in butter-slick crumbs and chocolate chips with the soles of my boots. It was as if I had lost control of my body completely. I was an animal, a savage, unable to do anything but howl and buck and thrash about.

Another time, while having the same old argument, this time in our bedroom, I flung my wedding band across the room and started packing an overnight bag. I jammed in my pajamas. A change of clothes. Toiletries. My phone. A book. My childhood E.T. doll. I fumbled with the zipper on my bag, partially blinded by my tears, snuffling mucus back up my nose so that it dripped down the back of my throat. But when I tried to leave the room, Michael blocked me.

"We should talk about this," Michael said, suddenly calm and rational and attentive now that I was on the verge of walking out the door.

"*I'm done talking!*" I screamed. Well, that or something equally melodramatic. My breakdowns made me revert to angsty teenager slash rabid dog every time they took over.

There was a scuffle. More screaming. More snot. Lots and lots of snot. Michael eventually wrestled me to the bed and lay on top of me like a weighted blanket until I finally burnt through all my angry energy and crumpled into myself, limp. Michael had always been the voice of reason, the counterpoint to my crazy, but as he marinated in his own unhappiness and disappointment, it was becoming more difficult for him to play this part.

During the day, when he was at work, I thought about what life might be like without him. What would become of me? Would I have to move back in with my parents, even though they had already converted my childhood bedroom into a home office? Would I have to return to corporate life in order to afford my own apartment? Would I have to wade back into the murky waters of online dating? Would I even be able to find someone I could be with the way I was with Michael? Easy? Honest? Comfortable? Troubled by this last train of thought, I turned back to logistics. Would I be able to keep the cat we adopted together? Would he be more likely to give up the cat if I let him keep all of the wedding gifts? The silverware? The pots and pans? The two different sets of wine glasses, the ones with cherry blossoms etched into their sides?

One day I wrote him a letter, trying to convey what I had been unable to convey in conversation. "I feel as if I'm your lowest priority," I wrote, "and that, frankly, you'd rather spend time with anyone—or anything— other than me." I wrote that I couldn't go on like this, and that I thought we should find a couples' therapist.

Two excruciating hours later, I got his response. "We aren't a good match," it began, and I was immediately queasy. "I thought we were, and maybe we were a better match in the past, but it's very clear this isn't true. Or at least I don't feel it's true anymore."

He suggested a trial separation.

I spent the rest of the work day in bed, crying, not crying, crying again. When I wasn't crying, I was frantically trying to think of a way to convince Michael that our marriage was worth working on, and that we were still good together. That we hadn't actually changed. That we were still the same people we'd each fallen in love with. When I lapsed back into tears, I thought of my mother and of how I wished she were there. I considered calling her, but I held off. Telling her would make it real, and I still couldn't believe that any of this was real. I waited for Michael to come home, hopeful that once we were in the same room he would realize he was being ridiculous. When he finally got home, I was still in bed. He stood in the doorway to our bedroom, looking at me, clearly already resigned to the end of our marriage. I sat up, crisscrossing my legs. He sat down next to me and drew his knees into his chest, hugging them close. "Well . . ." he said, and he stopped, glancing at me nervously. I took a breath and sighed it out.

We covered a lot of ground that evening, discussing everything that had felt broken in our relationship for the past few months. I explained why I was so upset about the late nights he spent in the city. I told him how hurtful it was that he oftentimes failed to tell me he wasn't coming straight home from work. "You have a spouse to come home to!" I said. "Do you even want to be married?"

"I don't know," he said. "Maybe I don't."

My tears dried up and my chest tightened. "You're

not leaving me because you're going through a mid-life crisis at the age of thirty-one," I said. "I'm not letting you do that."

He threw his hands up in the air. "I just feel as if marriage should be easier," he said. "We shouldn't have to compromise this much."

I couldn't believe what I was hearing. My nostrils flared, and my eyebrows shot toward my hairline. "That's what marriage is!" I said. "Marriage is about compromise! It isn't about finding your carbon copy. It isn't about finding your soul mate." I flapped my hands around in the air, trying to somehow convey the vast complexity of marriage, of a relationship that was intended to last the entirety of two people's lives. "It's about realizing you love someone, and deciding that you choose them," I tried to explain. "You choose *them* to spend the rest of your life with. It's about realizing that, and then working your ass off to make it work!"

My voice broke and I began to sob. He looked at me helplessly and then pulled me into his chest. I felt desperate in that moment and began bargaining for our marriage, telling him of all the ways I could change if it meant he would stay.

Finally, he suggested we sleep. I was a rag, twisted and wrung out and limp, and it felt good to slip beneath the covers and let my limbs go heavy. As he turned out his bedside lamp and lay down beside me, I curled into him, grasping, hysterical. He turned toward me, and we clutched at each other, my tears hot and steady as we had sex, three times in quick succession. It seemed somehow another betrayal—my body's ability to open itself up to the person who had just hurt me the most. But somewhere in there, Michael held me close and promised he wouldn't leave me. Mutual exhaustion eventually pulled us both toward asleep.

In the weeks after that, he kept flipping back and forth between being committed to our marriage and halfway out the door. "I'm not going to leave you," he'd insist while we were out on what was supposed to be a date, meant to bring us closer again. Then the next night, over wine and takeout Chinese and the latest crime procedural, he would change his mind. "I don't think we're a good match for each other. I just don't know . . ." he'd say. And I would break down all over again, turning into a sobbing, snotty mess, which would in turn cause him to lose his resolve. He'd again insist that we were okay. We'd end up in the bedroom, holding each other desperately, almost as if the only thing that could save us was to meld into each other's bodies, to become one. Afterwards, I'd feel used and confused by Michael's whipsawing desires. For months, I felt exhausted by my inability to know what was coming and relax into it.

Looking back on that time, Michael insists he did want to save our marriage, but needed to know that I wanted to as well. But how could either of us have known what the other was thinking? We were each wrapped up in our own problems and, even as each of us yearned to feel loved by the other, we were simultaneously pushing each other away.

It took some time to come back from that. Faced with the dissolution of our marriage, I gave the both of us homework, not sure how else to handle the situation.

First, we wrote Love Lists, identifying everything we loved about each other, reminding ourselves of why we were in the relationship in the first place. I wrote about his biceps, his sense of humor, and the way he was able to make me feel safe. I wrote about how grateful I was that he had always been open to trying *anything* with me. That he was so willing to do whatever it took to support my writing, even as it exposed his own life to the wider world. He wrote about my eyes, my laugh, and, I quote, "12. boobs." He wrote about my talent and ambition, and the way we could be our unfiltered selves with each other. "You had me write a love list," he wrote, "and it makes me love you more."

We also shared everything we hated, cognizant that we had to work on changing the things that were making us unhappy. Armed with this information, we scheduled time with a therapist—both individually and jointly—and learned how we might be better spouses to each other. Using reflective listening to explain our feelings to each other—our hurts—we were able to develop empathy for one another, to understand what the other person was going through instead of being stuck in the constant loop of negativity occurring in our own heads. This process helped me to fall in love with Michael all over again. If he sensed that I was getting flustered about something, he'd hold up a hand, say, "I think this is a good time for us to do some reflective listening." We would sit next to each other in bed, facing each other, and take turns. "When you push for me to go out with you and your friends," I might say, "even though I'm not in the mood, it makes me feel as if you don't know me. That you don't care about my anxiety." He'd repeat my words back to me, showing that he'd heard them and understood where I was coming from. And then he'd share his point of view. "When you don't try to connect with my friends," he'd say, "I feel as if you don't really want to be a part of my life. To know the people who are important to me." I'd, in turn, acknowledge the validity of his feelings, and we'd work on finding a solution that worked for the both of us. In this way, we slowly became a team again.

Amazingly, after a few months of this hard work, our marriage began to feel stronger than it ever had before. Not that things were perfect. We still grappled with how to handle our mismatched libidos, our sometimes-mismatched desires, our sadness and disappointment over the things in our life that were not going according to plan. But even where we disagreed, we were able to approach these problems as two people who still loved and respected each other.

When we got to that point—safe, stable, secure—we allowed ourselves to start thinking about a baby again. This time, however, we had to acknowledge that our bodies weren't doing their job, and that we might need help. And so, following another couple's recommendation, I made an appointment at a fertility center.

"How long have you two been trying?" the doctor asked us when the day of our appointment finally arrived, and we were seated before her expansive desk.

"About one and a half years," I responded, self-consciously squeezing my hands into the pleather armrests of my chair. I chose not to mention our small hiatus. "Is it too soon for us to be worried?"

"One and a half years? No, this is a good time to start considering other options. Typically, conception happens within the first year of trying, assuming there are no health complications." She passed each of us a folder filled with printouts that contained information on hormone treatments and IUI and IVF. I opened mine and began flipping through the pages as she explained all of the things that could affect a couple's ability to conceive naturally, and all of the tests that could be done to pinpoint such problems. "And if none of those tests yield any answers," she said, "we just assume the ovaries are underperforming." She looked at me apologetically. "There's really no good way to test for that, though. It's more a process of elimination."

I nodded my head, surprisingly untroubled by this, more relieved at finally being in the hands of fertility specialists. My body was underperforming. What else was new? But with the fertility specialists' battery of tests and their list of treatment options, surely we would get the answers we needed. And once we did, we'd know what to do. We'd have a plan. We'd know how to fix me. I wouldn't feel so powerless anymore.

With a renewed sense of optimism, I immediately began making my way through the list of tests, first going to a lab five minutes from home for blood work. This is when I realized this process might not be as cut-and-dry as I'd hoped.

"Relax," the phlebotomy technician hissed at me, her lips a tight gash across her face as I sat in one of those chairs with an adjustable armrest, staring at the smooth blankness of my inner arm. She smacked the inside of my elbow with the index and middle fingers of her right hand, trying to locate a vein, and furrowed her brow. "You're just making it harder for us," she said.

I sat there, breathing in and out, long and deep, through my nostrils, taking the slow, calming breaths I had learned at my yoga studio. My arm lay on the tray table attached to my armrest, completely relaxed because I had willed it so.

"Relax!" she barked at me again.

I looked into my lap and hated her.

The technician tied the elastic around my arm again, took aim with the needle, and slid it into my skin. She fiddled with it a bit, moving it around until my blood started creeping through the tube, toward an empty vial. I allowed myself to feel relief, for just a moment. Then the blood stopped, far short of its destination, and the technician's breath came out in a huff.

"You pregnant?" she asked me then, accusatory.

I swallowed. "No," I said, taking great care to muffle the bite in that one word. "I'm trying to figure out why I can't get pregnant."

Another tech tried, also without any luck. "Stop tensing up," she snapped at me, and I willed my arm to relax, though it didn't feel tense at all. I continued to breathe. Breathe. Breathe.

When I left that day, we hadn't been able to get the necessary amount of blood drawn.

The HSG wasn't any more pleasant. Lying back on a table, my feet in stirrups and an oversized paper towel covering my torso and upper body, as iodine squirted up through my cervix, I experienced intense cramping. Once again, I was forced to focus desperately on my breath for five endless minutes.

When it was over, they said everything looked good.

"Well, that's good, right?" asked my husband as we left the hospital.

I was quiet for a few moments as we made our way to the car. I wasn't sure how to respond. After all, we still didn't have any answers.

"Is it?" I finally asked.

One day, I drove my mom to an appointment to get bodywork done. The appointment took place in the sunroom of the practitioner's home, just off the living room. Waiting on the couch curled up with a book, I was eventually joined by the bodyworker's husband: someone I had seen in the past for both homeopathy and hypnotherapy. After a bit of small talk, I mentioned that my husband and I were trying to have a baby.

"There is no try," he said to me, an all-knowing smile on his face. "There is only making love."

My fingertips curled into the cover of the book I had been reading, my nails scratching furrows across the paper. It had been at least two years since I stopped taking my birth control pills. Two years since we started "making love" in earnest, at a frequency higher than at any other time in our marriage. Obviously, creating a child out of the union of our two bodies wasn't as simple as making love.

I swallowed the urge to punch him in the face.

We eventually began a round of IUI.

My husband volunteered to inject me with the necessary medication—intended to improve follicle growth—every night, his primary qualification being the fact that he shoved pills down two of our cats' throats every morning. This made him the most medically experienced person in the house.

Despite these qualifications, however, I cried the first time he prepared to inject me. Eventually, we put a sleep mask over my eyes so I couldn't see the needle coming closer to my exposed belly. When he made the injection, I barely felt a thing. Still, I insisted on wearing the sleep mask every night after that. I couldn't bring myself to watch.

In addition to the nightly injections, I woke up at 5 a.m. every other day to go into the fertility center for blood work and ultrasounds. These regular appointments left me exhausted and cranky . . . even more so on the days when the lab technicians struggled to find my veins.

I prepared for these visits by packing a bag with breakfast bars, a large water bottle, and two of my own stress balls. As I sat in the waiting room, awaiting my turn under the needle, I would gulp water, try to be subtle about the granola bar I was picking at, and work a stress ball in each hand so as to get my blood pumping.

When I finally walked into the back room, loaded down like a pack mule and still flexing my arm muscles, the lab techs would find my preparedness amusing.

Then they would try to find a vein.

Eventually, it was time for artificial insemination and, several days later, a pregnancy test. They called us at home several hours after the test.

"I'm sorry. You're not pregnant," the nurse said, and I swallowed once before responding.

"Oh, well. What can you do?" I said, fighting to keep my voice steady. "I guess we'll just have to try again."

I clicked the "off" button on the cordless and placed it beside me. I looked at my husband. He looked at me.

I burst into tears and he put his arms around me, rocking me back and forth. Snot gathered at my nostrils and tears soaked my collar.

"They told us it might not work the first time," he murmured into my ear. "We'll just try again next month."

We did. It didn't work then, either.

I was frustrated. The urologist my husband had first seen—a urologist the doctor at the fertility center had recommended—had told Michael that his sperm count wasn't fantastic, but that it was still good enough for us to go forward with the IUI. The doctors at the center, however, at both times of insemination, commented on the fact that Michael's count still wasn't optimal. *Why are we even doing this, then?* I wanted to know. *Why are you forcing me to go through with this if it's unlikely to work? Why are the fertility doctors and the urologist telling us two different things?*

When we first saw this urologist, after waiting for months to get a spot on his schedule, I thought his filled-to-the-brim schedule was a good sign. But since then, I decided I didn't like the guy. He seemed unresponsive. It took months to secure follow-up appointments. And he seemed disinterested in giving us any tips on how to boost Michael's count. After the second round of IUI failed us, I sought out recommendations for a new urologist.

The one we eventually chose was able to see us right away. Once again, we found ourselves seated across from yet another doctor hiding behind yet another long, gleaming desk. Again, we walked our way through our medical history. Then the doctor explained to us the results of the semen analysis he'd already done on Michael. "It's not necessarily that the count is low," he said. "The problem seems to be that there's an elevated number of white blood cells mixed in with the seminal fluid. These white blood cells can weaken the sperm."

He turned to Michael and began asking him about his dietary habits, his alcohol consumption. "Do you smoke?" he asked. I looked at Michael. He looked uncomfortable. He'd been a smoker when we met, and I'd made it clear that I had no interest in dating smokers. Since then, he allegedly kicked the habit.

"Yes," he said. He looked into his lap, his hands clasped tightly together. "Not regularly, but sometimes. Could that have caused this?"

I felt my face get hot; my jaw tightened. The doctor glanced at me. "It very well may have," he said and then, to me, "I assume this is the first you're hearing of this."

"Yes. It is," I said, taking great effort to keep my voice even. "Is there something that can be done about this?"

"You should stop smoking," the doctor said to Michael. I glared at him out of the corner of my eye, grinding my teeth. "Also, there's an antibiotic I can prescribe that should help. You'll have to take it for six months at which point we would do another semen analysis. When that happens, we can determine whether or not your count has improved enough to proceed with IUI or, more likely, IVF."

I sucked a breath in. I'd been hoping to avoid the more expensive IVF procedure, especially since we'd already paid for IUI twice, and were still unable to sell our condo. But what choice did we have? I had wanted to be a mother for just about as long as I'd wanted to be anything—since I started thinking about the future at all. I would do whatever I had to. IVF. Sperm donation. Adoption. Whatever it took.

I walked out of there grimly relieved that, once again, we had a plan. Still, I was silent as we made our way to the car. When we slid into our seats and slammed the doors shut, I just sat there, staring at the fuel gauge on the dashboard. Finally, with an intake of breath, I turned to Michael. "This entire time," I said, "I've been getting stuck with needles and waking up early for regular monitoring and having things stuck up my vagina. This entire time, I've been cutting back on coffee and avoiding booze. This entire time, I've been jumping through hoops, and it's been you." I paused and swallowed. "It's been you," I said again. "You've been jeopardizing our chance to have a baby. You've been lying to me and it's ruined everything."

I looked down, trying to blink away tears. I looked back up at him. "How could you do this?"

He stared down into his lap, aware that this new thing between us could destroy everything we worked to rebuild over the preceding months. "I've been under a lot of stress at work," he said. "I've been unhappy there. I *did* quit smoking," he assured me, finally looking me in the eye, "for a long time. But lately, I've been using it to cope."

We sat there in silence so I could absorb this new information. I grasped toward understanding, grasped for all the communication tools we developed in order to save our marriage; I grasped toward empathy.

There's nothing to be done about it, I finally told myself. *We can only move forward.*

I wasn't used to feeling so powerless. I was the type of person who identified problems, pinpointed possible solutions, developed plans, and took action. Being unable to control this one, important thing—with my ovulation trackers, with all of my best-laid plans, even with medical procedures—was maddening. It was yet another betrayal, this time by both of our bodies. And things never seemed to get any easier.

In the months Michael was taking his antibiotics, we turned toward the things we thought we *could* control. We were still unable to sell our condo, but we finally had enough money to purchase a house anyway. We began our search for a renter and had our realtor show us houses. Then, just as we found a house to bid on, Michael lost his job due to downsizing.

We bid anyway, as Michael felt certain he could get a new job in short order. Luckily, he was right, but the house we bid on was a short sale, which promised a long, drawn out process of at least six months during which we would be at the complete mercy of the bank.

As we waited it out, Michael turned his thoughts toward sex, and I remained sick with worry at what might happen with the short sale. Because the proportion of sperm to white blood cells in his system was slowly improving, Michael insisted we keep trying to conceive naturally. "Let's make a baby tonight," he'd say, wiggling his hips mock-seductively.

I wasn't interested. I was too busy feeling stressed out. In fact, I'd get angry, accusing him of trying to manipulate me, of trying to use my desire for a baby as a means of fulfilling his desire to get off. I knew this was unfair. I knew he wanted a baby just as much as I did. But after having scheduled baby-making sex for so long—and doing two rounds of IUI on top of that—I truly believed it was impossible for us to conceive naturally, and I found it hard to trust that he might think otherwise. I didn't like considering the possibility that he was using the dangling carrot of conception to get into my pants.

Finally, Michael got another semen analysis done, and we were told we could go forward with IVF. The only problem this time was that where his previous health insurance plan would have covered the procedure in full, his new employer wouldn't cover a single cent. We would have to pay eighteen thousand dollars fully out of pocket. We didn't have that kind of money, especially now that we had two mortgages to contend with. The house we bid on was finally ours, and though we had found a renter for our condo, we weren't breaking even with the monthly rent. Instead, we were losing several hundred dollars every month, a loss we determined we could handle before learning about both the cost of IVF and the limitations of our health insurance. The only thing we could do was put off the procedure again while we saved up the money we needed.

During this excruciating period of limbo, Michael continued taking the antibiotics. He liked to joke that he was building up super sperm. And perhaps he was. When we were finally able to afford IVF, he had yet another semen analysis done. The results were so positive that the doctors thought it was worth trying the cheaper IUI again—this time without the nightly injections I typically endured. His count was just that good. For the first time in a long time—though only cautiously—I allowed myself to feel hope. Excitement, even. I waited for my next menstruation to start so we could once again move forward. So we could start the process all over again.

"Did you get your period today?" Michael asked, on the exact day it was due.

"No," I told him, "but it's typically a few days late."

"Did you get your period today?" he asked the next day.

"No," I said, "but that's normal."

"Did you get your period today?" he asked the next day, and then two days after that.

"I'm going to slap you," I said.

Though I might have allowed myself to hope again about pregnancy in general, that hope was firmly connected to the IUI process. I still didn't believe we could conceive without a little extra push from the medical establishment.

That weekend, we had a party at our place. I drank from the giant crystal bowl of mimosa punch placed in the center of our dining room table, enough to be pleasantly tipsy as I milled about the crowd of fifty-odd people. For at least a few hours, I didn't think about menstruation. About infertility. About babies.

For a few hours, I didn't think, period.

The next day, my mother convinced me to try an at-home pregnancy test. I was a week late and had been complaining about feeling run down. All of the tests I initially received with my boxes of fertility-friendly lube had long since expired, so Michael and I made a late-night run to the corner CVS. So overwhelmed were we by the variety of options that I had to ask the pharmacist for advice.

Upon returning home, I opened up the box to read through the instructions while simultaneously chugging water. The instructions seemed dauntingly complex. I worried about not keeping the pee stick perfectly horizontal. I worried about waiting too long or not long enough for the results. I worried that the results would be unclear because, according to the instructions, that was possible, too.

Eventually, I locked myself in the bathroom, pulled down my pants, and did my business. I laid the stick carefully down on the tiled floor, on top of a small square of toilet paper, taking great pains to keep it horizontal at all times. I stepped clear of the toilet, pulled up my pants, closed the lid, and sat back down to wait, my forearms on my thighs, my head hanging down between my knees. There was a churning in my gut, and my hands shook slightly.

Sooner than I expected, black markings popped up on the screen. I leaned closer. It said: **YES**.

I picked up the stick and, using the tissue, removed every trace of pee from its surface, looking at it again.

YES.

I checked again.

It still said **YES**.

"How's it going in there?" asked Michael, right outside the door.

I held the stick in my hand. My voice was uncertain. "I think we might be pregnant?"

"What?"

I quietly unlocked and opened the bathroom door. I showed Michael the pregnancy test. "Could this be true?" I said. I stumbled about our kitchen in a daze, holding the pregnancy test before me. "Oh my god," I said. My hands still shook.

I kept checking the test again and again, expecting the results to change. To fade away, perhaps. To switch to **NO**. I placed the test inside a plastic baggie and put it aside. I still thought the results might change.

Perhaps they would switch to something crueler, like **LOL, J/K!**, I thought. I kept retrieving the bag, peering through the plastic at the little black **YES**. I still couldn't allow myself to believe it.

When I called my mom, I told her that—according to the pee stick, at least—I was probably pregnant. "I'm so happy for you," she said, her voice thin with emotion, and immediately burst into tears.

"Me too," I said, and immediately burst into tears as well.

Michael was giggly and giddy and all wound up as he walked over and put his arms around me. Standing there in the middle of our kitchen, he rocked me back and forth. Snot gathered at my nostrils and tears soaked my collar. His shirt became wet.

We stood there for a long time, him rubbing my back, me sniffling.

Afterward, I still kept checking the tiny screen on

the test to make sure nothing had changed. I couldn't foresee what my future held: the shame I'd feel in regard to my postpartum depression due to the fact that I'd wanted this for so long . . . the sense of overwhelm I would feel as a work-at-home mother . . . the heart-exploding love I would feel despite all of this.

I only knew that my dreams were finally coming true.

8 YOU ARE NOT ALONE

In 2010, flibanserin—touted as the female Viagra—was rejected by the Food and Drug Administration (FDA) for the first time. In 2013, it was rejected again. In January 2014, the FDA requested even further safety testing. The primary reason? The risks (and the side effects, such as nausea, dizziness, and drowsiness) were considered greater than the reward.[5]

Still, on February 27, 2015, Sprout Pharmaceuticals, which had taken charge of the drug's development, announced that it had submitted a New Drug Application (NDA) to the FDA. Though initially developed as an antidepressant, flibanserin was allegedly found to boost libido.[6] On the evening of Tuesday, August 18, 2015, flibanserin— a nonhormonal pill developed to

5   Sarah Kaplan. "The Fight for a 'female Viagra'." *The Washington Post*. June 1, 2015.

6   Sprout Pharmaceuticals. "Sprout Pharmaceuticals Resubmits Flibanserin New Drug Application For The Treatment Of Hypoactive Sexual Desire Disorder In Premenopausal Women. Sprout Pharmaceuticals, Inc." Sprout Pharmaceuticals Inc. February 17, 2015.

treat Hypoactive Sexual Desire Disorder (HSDD) in premenopausal women, and which would need to be taken daily—was approved by the FDA.[7]

There are those—especially women with lackluster libidos—who think it's about damn time. Women's sexual health advocacy group Even the Score, for example, pointed out at the time that there were already twenty-six government-approved drugs made available to treat sexual dysfunction in men. They accused the FDA of being sexist because of the lack of a comparable drug for women.[8] And they were thrilled that an FDA advisory committee finally voted to recommend approval of flibanserin.[9]

So why haven't sexual health care providers collectively lost their shit over flibanserin, throwing confetti into the air and twerking around their offices?

For one thing, if we're going to get technical, we can't *really* develop a female version of Viagra, because the problems of erectile dysfunction (ED) and HSDD are very different. ED is primarily a mechanical issue, not an issue of desire, and Viagra is meant to increase blood flow to the genitals that may be hindered by circulatory system problems.

Women's desire is another thing entirely: a complex confluence of circumstances that includes our hormones, our brain chemistry, our cultural expectations, and a

---

7   Brigid Schulte and Brady Dennis. "FDA Approves Controversial Drug for Women with Low Sex Drives." *The Washington Post.* August 18, 2015. Accessed August 19, 2015.

8   "The Problem." Even The Score. Accessed July 30, 2015.

9   Ellie Shechet. "FDA Advisory Committee Approves 'Female Viagra' Drug ." Jezebel. June 5, 2015.

barrage of interior questions in reference to whether or not we did the laundry (or the food shopping, or that work task, or that diaper change) yet. Something this multifaceted is much more difficult to manage than what can be accomplished by simply popping a pill every night before bed.

Which is why flibanserin has taken so long to hustle its way into existence. The drug has to work in a completely different way than Viagra, targeting women's brains in order to counteract all the chaos that may be suppressing our desire to get it on. It has to increase the effects of desire-enhancing chemicals such as dopamine while simultaneously decreasing the impact of inhibitors such as serotonin.[10]

And in fact, according to research published in the *Journal of Sexual Medicine,* after studying more than eleven thousand women who tried taking flibanserin for their HPDD, there was a 37 percent reported increase in desire among the study's participants.[11]

This is all well and good, but there was a second issue causing skepticism among many sexologists at the time flibanserin was approved, the very people Sprout Pharmaceuticals would hope to have on its side: the fact that the pharmaceutical industry seemed to be pathologizing women's sexuality rather than supporting it. After all, when you identify as someone who has low

---

10 Diane Kelly. "Here's How That New Sex Pill for Women Actually Works." Throb. June 29, 2015.

11 Molly Katz, Leonard R. Derogatis, Ronald Ackerman, Parke Hedges, Lynna Lesko, Miguel Garcia, and Michael Sand. "Efficacy of Flibanserin in Women with Hypoactive Sexual Desire Disorder: Results from the BEGONIA Trial." *The Journal of Sexual Medicine* 10, no. 7 (2013): 1807–815. doi:10.1111/jsm.12189.

sexual desire, or you diagnose someone with low sexual desire, what does that even mean? How much desire *should* you be feeling? Low in relation to whom?

In June of 2010, I was asking myself the same question, as I was still experiencing much lower levels of desire than my husband. I pre-gamed for sex by warming myself up with the latest vibrator, willing my clitoris to wake the eff up so I could enjoy moderately pleasurable intercourse without the use of multiple gallons of lube. I did this tucked under the covers, wrist aching from the pressure and the strain. All the while, my husband prepared himself in the bathroom across the hall, shaving away his stubble because he knew I hated the way it felt rubbing against my chin and my lips. I would press the vibrator harder through the lips of my vulva as one or more of my cats sat at the foot of my bed, staring at me. *Hurry up!* I told my clitoris, my eyes squinting in concentration. *Let's have just one orgasm before he gets here!*

During this time, I read books about pleasure and libido and orgasms, building up a body of research that allowed me to write listicles for lifestyle sites such as YourTango and The Frisky and The Date Report. Ironically, I was writing articles on how to do two things I had never been able to do for myself: boost your libido and have even better orgasms.

"Feeling appreciated will most likely make him want to show his appreciation, too, making your days a non-stop love-fest," I wrote in a perky tone, insinuating that I had experienced at least one, full-day, nonstop love-fest of my own (I hadn't). In suggesting partner yoga as a means of striking a spark, I wrote "a level of intimacy arises that may be conducive to getting flexible in the bedroom later on." In reality, my husband confessed to me that he had spent the entirety of our first partner yoga class together trying to hold in his farts.

Aside from my career as a writer of wishful thinking, I also managed various content partnerships with similar lifestyle sites that, like YourTango, dabbled in blog posts and personal essays about love, sex, and relationships. One day, my contact at one of these sites asked me if I would be interested in writing a sex advice column for them. Making it clear that I myself was not an expert, but that I could certainly use the research of actual experts in combination with my own anecdotal evidence as a means of getting the job done, I accepted the gig.

I spent the next six months combing through emails, writing up columns on incompatible sex drives, sex toys in the context of partner sex, painful sex, and butt play. I shared stories of my own waning libido and the frustration I felt when my gynecologist seemed unconcerned with the pain I reported having during intercourse. I shared tips I had come across from various sexuality professionals. More than anything, I tried to express empathy over infinite wisdom.

I tried to cover as wide a range of topics as possible in my column, but there were still so many emails I never got the chance to respond to. So many questions. So many pleas for help. The guilt I felt over this haunted me. I wanted to be able to fix everyone's problems almost as much as I wanted to fix my own.

And even as I filed my columns, I was never sure that the response I had given was the right one. Who was I to tell someone that this or that thing would change their lives, would make everything all better? I could only share what I had experienced myself, and what I had gleaned from numerous sexuality professionals through their books and research: a collection of mostly obvious and bland pieces of general advice that had been regurgitated over and over again across the Internet until, at some point, they had become meaningless.

That same year, Ian Kerner, a sex counselor I once interviewed for a story in *Time Out New York,* reached out to ask if I would be interested in coauthoring an e-book with him for his new sex education site, Good in Bed. Kerner was the author of the popular *She Comes First,* a book I had reviewed for the Sex Herald, and which I then gave to my husband to read. The fact that he asked me, of all people, to collaborate with him on a new book seemed somewhat mind-boggling.

Regardless, I threw myself into this new challenge and, as I continued writing my way through my various Sex with Steph columns, I also worked with Ian Kerner, PhD to create *52 Weeks of Amazing Sex*. The basic premise behind the book was that romantic partners should aim to have sex with each other at least once a week in order to maintain optimal levels of intimacy within the relationship. To aid in this, we came up with fifty-two suggestions—one for each week of the year— that would challenge couples to experiment with the various permutations of what sex is and can be, enabling them to keep things exciting and, by extension, keep the spark in their relationships glowing white hot.

As I wrote up the content for each of those fifty-two weeks, I considered that it could be beneficial for

Michael and me to also experiment with all of the suggestions in *52 Weeks*. At that point in our relationship, however, we were having sex only once every few months. The thought of increasing the frequency of our physical intimacy that suddenly and drastically was daunting.

Aside from the guilt I felt in knowing that Michael wanted sex far more often than I did, I didn't miss it for myself. I wasn't humping pillows and penetrating myself with my vibrator in horny, unfulfilled desperation. What we were doing, as sparse as it might seem to others, felt like . . . enough.

Did that mean there was something wrong with me? That I was broken? Were we all broken—all the men and women who had written in to me for advice, all the people who eventually downloaded *52 Weeks of Amazing Sex* in droves? Were we *all* suffering from various forms of sexual dysfunction?

In 1964, sex researchers William Masters and Virginia Johnson developed the four-phase model of sexual response: 1. Excitement. 2. Plateau. 3. Orgasm. 4. Resolution. According to Emily Nagoski, PhD in her book *Come As You Are,* this model quickly became the basis for defining both sexual health and sexual problems—sexual "dysfunctions," if you will—establishing a norm of sorts for sexual behavior and allowing clinicians to compare their clients' experiences to what they felt *should* be happening in the bedroom.[12]

---

12 Emily Nagoski. *Come as You Are: The Surprising New Science That Will Transform Your Sex Life.* New York: Simon & Schuster, 2015.

In the 1970s, psychotherapist Helen Singer Kaplan, MD, PhD developed her triphasic model after discovering that the concept of sexual desire—or lust—was missing from the already existing and dominant theory of sexual response. By contrast, her model *began* with desire, which was then followed by arousal, and ended in orgasm. Kaplan felt that one must be psychologically interested in sex before the body could adequately respond to sexual overtures. The acknowledgment of one's longing for intimacy, and how it might affect arousal, was an important one. Still, though her model rectified weaknesses in the preceding model, it presumed that desire always came first, whether for men or for women, and it painted a picture of goal-oriented sex that always ended in orgasm.

In 2001, Rosemary Basson, MD published a paper in the *Journal of Sex & Marital Therapy*[13] that began to lay out the ways in which female sexual desire worked differently than male sexual desire. Her descriptions of the human sex-response cycles for both men and women showed that, while men often experienced desire first, which then led them to make an overture of sex before even having an erection, women usually experienced desire only after first being physically aroused. This meant that you could wait possibly forever for a woman to find herself "in the mood" for sex. Instead, if you really wanted to have sex with your female partner, the best course of action would be to actively stimulate her, making her think *Ooh, that felt*

---

13 Rosemary Basson. "Human Sex-Response Cycles." *Journal of Sex & Marital Therapy*, no. 27 (2001): 33–43.

good. It would be fun to do more of that. Maybe we should get it on.

I'm simplifying of course, but Basson's work began to help many people understand, some of them for the first time, that women's experience of desire could be far more complex than men's. And not only that, but the inherent complexity of the sexual response cycle in women meant that those who weren't experiencing automatic desire (and, rather, were experiencing only responsive desire) were behaving in completely normal and expected ways. I should note here that this is also a generalization. Both men and women are capable of experiencing both automatic and responsive desire; it's just that, statistically, the numbers tend to lean toward one direction or the other.

There are those, however, who have found the blazing light of truth in a model developed in the late 1990s by Erick Janssen and John Bancroft of the Kinsey Institute: the dual control model.[14] In *Come As You Are,* Nagoski extols its virtues, explaining how it addresses not just what happens during arousal, but also everything that might affect how and when it happens. How does it work? Basically, the dual control model acknowledges that our sexual response system, much like every other part of the central nervous system, operates in an ever-shifting tug of war between activation and inhibition. Our sexual excitation system—the activation part of the equation, which Nagoski refers to as our sexual accelerator—

---

14 "The Dual-Control Model: The Role of Sexual Inhibition & Excitation in Sexual Arousal and Behavior." In *The Psychophysiology of Sex*, edited by Erick Janssen, 197–222. Bloomington, Indiana: Indiana University Press, 2007.

notices sexually relevant information in our environment and nudges us to get it on. Some examples of sexually relevant information include the way your partner smells right out of the shower, how he looks freshly shaved, and the warm fuzzies you feel when he does something especially thoughtful for you, unsolicited. On the flip side, the sexual inhibition system—the brakes—notices all the reasons there might be for not engaging in sexy time. Examples include body image issues, a traumatic sexual history, feelings of obligation and their attendant feelings of resentment, performance anxiety, depression, anxiety, stress . . . basically all of the things I tended to be grappling with on any given day. This tug of war is ongoing and can have a huge bearing on whether or not you choose to dive into bed with your partner or turn away from him when he puts the moves on you.

When I first read about this model, I began to understand how everything from my rapidly expanding to-do list to the dismal state of my pedicure might turn me off of the idea of sex entirely. It was no wonder I was never in the mood.

Still, the existence and supposed validity of various types of female sexual dysfunction had, by this point, been pretty well entrenched in the public consciousness. And while there were some forms of sexual dysfunction that had their basis in actual, physiological issues of functionality (such as vaginismus, a painful, spasmodic contraction of the vagina in response to physical contact or pressure), diagnoses such as that of HSDD were a little bit tougher to pin down.

The pathologization, and ensuing medicalization, of female sexuality started in the 1930s when those working in the field of psychoanalysis found themselves preoccupied with the difficulties inherent in female sexuality, most common among them being "frigidity."[15] And while some time passed before various forms of sexual dysfunction disorders were officially acknowledged in the most respected of clinical texts, they were finally added to the *Diagnostic and Statistical Manual of Mental Disorders (DSM)*—a manual used for diagnostic purposes by many clinical professionals—in 1980. This section of the *DSM* was revised in 1987 and 1994, expanded to include struggles with issues such as the sexual response cycle and painful intercourse.

A more recent edition of the *DSM* also made reference to "hypoactive sexual desire disorder, sexual aversion disorder, sexual arousal disorder, orgasmic disorder, dyspareunia, vaginismus, and sexual dysfunctions caused by medical conditions, substance use, or other unspecified causes." And the fifth edition, issued in 2013, merged desire and arousal into a single entry known as female sexual interest/arousal disorder, or FSIAD. This update has drawn the ire of some critics, who have argued that desire and arousal are two very distinct aspects of female sexual response.

Similarly, the World Health Organization's (WHO) *International Statistical Classification of Diseases and Related Health Problems, 10th Revision*, defines sexual dysfunction as "people's inability to participate in sexual relationships as they wish." Specific diagnoses

---

15 Katherine Angel. "The History Of 'Female Sexual Dysfunction' As A Mental Disorder In The 20th Century." *Current Opinion in Psychiatry* 23, no. 6 (2010): 536–41.

mentioned in this particular manual include "lack or loss of desire, sexual aversion and lack of sexual enjoyment, vaginal dryness, markedly delayed or nonexistent orgasm, vaginismus and dyspareunia not attributable to physical problems, and excessive sexual drive."[16]

And there has been considerable research conducted on the topic as well. According to the *Los Angeles Times,* one of the most frequently cited studies analyzed data from a 1992 National Health and Social Life Survey.[17] Published in the *Journal of the American Medical Association* in 1999, the authors of this study reported that 43 percent of the women they surveyed experienced sexual dysfunction of one sort or another. And of that 43 percent, 22 percent cited low desire.[18] Interestingly, it was later revealed that the lead researcher on this study had ties to the pharmaceutical company Pfizer, the makers of Viagra.

This is only one of many examples in which studies showing high incidences of sexual dysfunction among the female population were found to be funded by pharmaceutical companies with high stakes in the results. For example, in 2005, Pfizer funded another survey, one that showed 63 percent of women had sexual dysfunction, and that testosterone and Viagra might be helpful.

---

16 R. A. Clay. "What Is 'Female Sexual Dysfunction'?" *Monitor on Psychology* 40, no. 4 (2009): 35.

17 Jessica Pauline Ogilvie. "Debate on Female Sexual Dysfunction Continues" *Los Angeles Times.* June 28, 2010. Accessed August 19, 2015.

18 E. O. Laumann, Anthony Paik, and Raymond C. Rosen. "Sexual Dysfunction in the United States: Prevalence and Predictors." *JAMA: The Journal of the American Medical Association* 281, no. 6 (1999): 537–44.

In 2006, Procter and Gamble, the makers of a testosterone patch for women, sponsored a survey showing that one in ten postmenopausal women had HSDD. And in 2008, Boehringer Ingelheim, the initial developers of flibanserin before Sprout Pharmaceuticals took over, sponsored a survey that also showed that one in ten women were looking for a libido-booster.[19] At the time, I know that I would have counted myself among them.

Other studies looking at the prevalence of female sexual dysfunction have produced more widely divergent results, showing that anywhere from less than 10 percent to more than 50 percent of women have low desire.

So where does the truth lie? How pervasive is the problem of female sexual dysfunction, and what is to be done about its encroaching spread throughout our bedrooms?

The truth is, there is no existing standard for what "normal" is and, as such, no hard and fast rule for what counts as "abnormal."

After the success of Viagra—a drug created to manage erectile dysfunction (ED)—the pharmaceutical industry was eager to create a similar market for sexual dysfunction drugs for women. Unfortunately, there was not yet a clearly defined medical diagnosis for a form of female sexual dysfunction that could be considered comparable to ED. Thus began the creation and shaping

---

19 Jeremy Laurence. "Female Sexual Dysfunction 'Invented by Drugs Industry'" *Belfast Telegraph*. January 10, 2010. Accessed August 19, 2015.

of the definitions for various desire and arousal disorders.

While definitions of sexual dysfunction specify that distress must be present in order for something to qualify as a disorder, the existence of such diagnoses themselves can prime women to feel that a problem exists.

No one really knows what it means to have normal levels of desire, arousal, or orgasm. There is no official metric for diagnosis, despite the many attempts over the years to measure desire and arousal. Because of this, some sexuality professionals accuse those in the pharmaceutical industry of medicalizing what, for many, are just the natural ups and downs of life. In Ray Moynihan, PhD's *Sex, Lies, and Pharmaceuticals*, for instance, Kinsey Institute research scientist Erick Janssen, PhD, is quoted as saying about the lack of clear measurement tools with which to define FSD: "It's like using a ruler without marks."

Many tools have been developed over the years in order to pinpoint what is normal when it comes to arousal and desire, and many studies have been conducted on the efficacy of these tools, but none of these studies have truly been able to encompass the complexity of female sexual response. This is because they overstate the importance of physical factors while continuing to ignore the psychological and social factors that can contribute to lower sexual functioning.

While researchers continue to develop new measurement tools, just as many sexologists maintain a focus on fighting back against the rapidly encroaching medicalization of women's sexuality. The New View Campaign, for example, was formed in 2000 as a grassroots network dedicated to challenging "the distorted and oversimplified messages about sexuality that the pharmaceutical industry relies on to sell its new drugs."[20] They have since pointed out that many classifications of female sexual desire follow the models of male sexual desire, which have since been shown to be inaccurate when applied to females. In 2012, *The Journal of Sex Research* published an entire issue devoted to the medicalization of sex.[21] And there are other researchers, among them Kristen Mark, PhD, MPH, who have pointed out that many reports of sexual satisfaction (or lack thereof) seem to be inextricably tied to their partner's satisfaction.[22] What does *this* mean when it comes to creating a barometer for "low" sexual desire?

It's now been about five years since I wrote my sex advice column, and since I coauthored *52 Weeks of Amazing Sex*. And as I think back on the slew of questions that slid their way into my email inbox, I can't help thinking that all of them, in one way or another, could be boiled down to one, simple question: Am I normal?

When so many people see fit to question their level of normality, it stands to reason that, while the arc of human sexuality contains many variations, just about all of us are within the realm of average. Ordinary. Commonplace. None of us need to be fixed, because none of us are broken.

---

20 New View Campaign. Accessed August 19, 2015. http://www .newviewcampaign.org/.

21 *The Journal of Sex Research* 49, no. 4 (2012).

22 Kristen Mark. "Self Reports of Sexual Satisfaction: Who Is The Self?" Kinsey Confidential. March 7, 2012. Accessed August 19, 2015.

Perhaps we just need to expand our definition of what sex is. What it can be. And to tell ourselves it's okay when we don't want it.

And perhaps we would all be better served by the assurance that we're far from alone, rather than being given a knee-jerk diagnosis and a questionable cure.

After being blocked from approval twice before, the most recent decision from the FDA to approve flibanserin doesn't seem to indicate any sense of confidence in the efficacy of the drug, or any sense of confidence that the risks that were initially deemed a concern have been sufficiently dealt with. In fact, flibanserin's approval comes with a long list of conditions that reflect the agency's concerns about the side effects, which include low blood pressure and fainting in patients who drink alcohol while taking the drug. And doctors are required to complete a training course before even being allowed to prescribe it.

"Because of a potentially serious interaction with alcohol, treatment with Addyi [the name under which flibanserin will now be marketed] will only be available through certified health care professionals and certified pharmacies," said Janet Woodcock, director of the FDA's Center for Drug Evaluation and Research, in a statement.[23] The FDA also recommended that women stop using the pill if they noticed no change in their libido after eight weeks.

The aforementioned advocacy group Even the Score

---

23 "FDA Approves First Treatment for Sexual Desire Disorder." U.S. Food and Drug Administration. August 18, 2015. http://www.fda .gov/NewsEvents/Newsroom/PressAnnouncements/ucm458734 .htm.

considers this to be a win for feminism. What's interesting is that Even the Score was formed by Sprout Pharmaceuticals in 2014 and is still partly funded by Sprout. And there are those who believe that the feminist angle concocted by Sprout and Even the Score and used to push the FDA to approve flibanserin was integral in this recent "win."[24]

So it seems that this is more of a win for the pharmaceutical industry than anything else. And a loss for women who continue to be inundated with messages telling them that if they don't want sex as much as their partner, or as much as our culture at large deems appropriate, there's something wrong with them.

Then again, Addyi had a poor showing in its first four weeks on the market. During that time, doctors wrote just 227 prescriptions for Addyi. By contrast, over the same period of time in 1998, more than half a million men got prescriptions for Viagra, according to data from IMS Health. Could it be that there is not as much demand for a libido-boosting pill as groups such as Even the Score would have us believe? Could it be that women realize the issue of libido is more complex than anything a pill could touch?

Even more importantly, what could be accomplished if funding were provided for research that focused on a more holistic approach to women's dissatisfaction with their sex lives? An approach that touched upon relational and cultural factors?

---

24 Azeen Ghorayshi. "How Big Pharma Used Feminism To Get The 'Female Viagra' Approved." BuzzFeed. August 18, 2015. Accessed August 19, 2015.

Lori Brotto, an associate professor in the Department of Obstetrics and Gynecology at the University of British Columbia, and a member of one of the committees that worked on updates to the most recent edition of the DSM, spoke to me about lopsided research funding for a piece I wrote for Undark. At the time, she noted that one of the reasons there's such a focus on medically-based treatments is because that's where the money is. "There's a bias in the kind of science that is getting done," she said.

If more attention were paid to the types of treatments sexologists like Brotto focus on—such as cognitive behavioral therapy (CBT), mindfulness exercises, and couples therapy—would we start to think about what women actually want from their sex lives versus what they're allegedly lacking?

When I first read Come As You Are, the realization that I was defining my own sexual health by how often I felt desire in relation to my husband walloped me upside the head and left me stunned. At the time, because of my role as social media manager for Ian Kerner's Good in Bed site, I had been tasked with organizing a Twitter Q+A with Nagoski. Doing my due diligence, I read the entire book so I could draw up a set of questions for the author.

I soon found myself dog-earing every other page of Nagoski's book, underlining passages on how we view our bodies, how sexual response tends to work differently for different segments of the population, and how traumatic experiences can inform future intimate relationships. I was fascinated by how scientists' theories about sexual response had evolved over the years. I took notes on how various cues in our environment could affect sexual response differently depending upon the context in which they were experienced. I highlighted an entire page on sexual violence and trauma and our bodies' fight/flight/freeze responses. I was more than halfway through the book when I came to the passage that changed everything. The one that finally gave me permission to release that internal image of myself as defective, dysfunctional, broken.

I was sitting in bed with Nagoski's book, my back propped up on a pile of pillows and yoga bolsters, Michael sleeping beside me, when I read several paragraphs about the lie behind the existence of "low" desire. "Problematic dynamics emerge," Nagoski wrote, "when the partners have different levels of desire *and* they believe that one person's desire is 'better' than the other person's." She went on to explain that the partner who wants sex more infrequently is often seen as in some way deficient, and that the partner with the higher level of desire is seen as "normal." Her underlying message, obviously, was that this was bullshit. I dog-eared the page because I found the concept interesting, and also empowering for women in general, but I wasn't really thinking about its ramifications on my own life. I continued reading.

"Don't just run, be a runner," wrote Nagoski several pages later. "Don't just have sex, be a deliciously erotic woman who is curious and playful about sex. If you run because you have to or you feel like you're supposed to, rather than because it's part of who you are, you won't run very far or very often, and you probably won't enjoy it much when you do. And if you have sex because you have to **or you feel like you're supposed to** [*emphasis mine*], you won't have much sex and you probably won't enjoy it when you do."

It hit me then: the ways in which I pushed myself to fulfill Michael's needs without considering my own. The way in which I'd been viewing his sex drive as the default, how I was supposed to be, when in fact—especially considering the prevalence of self-reported incidences of "low" libido—*I* could more accurately be defined as the normal one.

Not that the word "normal" had much meaning at all.

I clutched at my bedspread as the gears in my head turned, shifting to reframe the past fifteen years of my life. My eyes filled up and overflowed with tears, the words on the pages before me blurring. I had spent the past fifteen years trying to boost my libido to match someone else's desires, and I felt free knowing I didn't have to do it anymore. I had spent the past fifteen years shaping my career so that I could use it to bolster my own quest for a sexual "cure." How many other people were doing the same thing?

As my mind was being blown, Michael slept on, unawares. I ended up finishing the entire book that night, even as my eyes burned from exhaustion. Then I placed the book aside, slid beneath my covers, switched off my bedside lamp, and slept the sleep of the newly vindicated.

The next time Michael propositioned me, I pounced on the chance to share what I'd learned. "You want some of this?" he asked one night as we were changing into our pajamas. He was half kidding, yes, but also clearly hoping that I would pleasantly surprise him by ripping off my bra and leaping into bed.

"You know . . ." I said, which is maybe Michael's least favorite phrase alongside "I have to tell you something" and "there's something we need to discuss." I went for it anyway. "Just because I don't want to have sex as often as you do," I said, "it doesn't mean that there's something wrong with me."

"Uh huh," Michael said, with the understanding that we were clearly not about to have sex.

"I was reading about female sexual response," I continued, waving Nagoski's book in the air, "and it's completely normal for me not to be in the mood all the time. And I'd appreciate it if you could respect that."

"I do," Michael said, pulling on a T-shirt and scrubs in preparation for an evening without sex.

"And also," I continued, because I am a joy to live with when I'm on a tear about something, "I shouldn't actually be expected to be in the mood out of nowhere. There are *so many things* that can dampen libido. Stress. Exhaustion. Depression. I need a little help to get there. I wanna be *wooed*."

"Uh huh," Michael said.

And then we slid into bed—I with a new book and he with his iPad—and we did not have sex. Michael was disappointed, but at least he understood.

And as for me? For once, I didn't go into all of the usual emotional contortions: feeling pressured to feel desire, feeling guilty that I wasn't giving him what he wanted, feeling resentment that I had to feel pressured and guilty at all. For once, I felt at ease.

Still, respecting your partner's sexual drives goes

both ways, and I knew we had to find a way to compromise. A large part of Nagoski's book, after all, had been given over to the sexual brakes and accelerators, and I knew that pinpointing my own personal activators and inhibitors would provide me with the key to actually *enjoying* sex . . . not just finding ways to justify not having it.

Achieving (sexual) enlightenment is a process. And this one would require some additional trial and error. Fortunately, without the added pressure of all those outsized expectations I'd long been holding for myself, it became that much easier to focus on what brought me pleasure and on what turned me off. In time, sex became something I could sometimes enjoy, not something I had to speed-hump my way through out of obligation. And during that time—though my epiphany about out-of-sync libidos and the complexity of the sexual response cycle revealed to me that my entire career had been built upon a massive misperception—I continued to write about sexuality.

Except now, I wasn't writing to fix myself. Instead, I was writing to spread the gospel of truth. I was writing to tell those who'd long felt deficient that they could begin enjoying sex the way they actually wanted it. Not the way they felt they should.

I was writing to tell everyone: you're completely normal.

9 | THE WORD I CANNOT SAY

I see him across the room. And though we are in a noisy and crowded bar—karaoke in the back, drinkers up front, darts players scrunched in between—it is like being wiped out by a wave, head plunged into water, sounds muffled and watery, me sputtering, searching for sky, trying to breathe.

Five years before, I had loved him.

Five years before, he snatched away my virginity.

Five years.

There are still snippets of sound and sensation I can remember clearly.

I remember the dark of the rec room, the locked door at the top of the stairs, my toes flexing and sliding in the shag carpeting as we sat side by side on the couch. I remember laying back against a throw pillow, his mouth on mine, his fingers inside me, my hands on his back.

I remember him, just a shadow in the dark, and the sound of his mesh shorts whispering down his legs and pooling onto the carpet with a soft schloomp.

No, when he climbed on top of me, I didn't say "no" or "stop."

But I didn't say "yes," either. I only squeezed my thighs together, tight as I could, as he pressed himself against me, as he pressed himself inside me.

When he left that night, I cried for hours until my eyes were red and raw and my body was limp. But despite my visceral reaction to this incident, I stayed with him for four more months. Despite what he had done, I thought I still loved him. I thought our love was real in spite of the ways he hurt me over and over again. And perhaps most discouraging of all, I saw all of his behavior as something we could come back from. The way he claimed ownership of me—an ownership that superseded even my own rights to my body and to my life—were distressing, yes. But as unhappy as I was for so much of the time, I didn't look at the two of us and see an unhealthy relationship. That understanding only came later.

Seeing him across that room, five years later, is disorienting. I am surrounded by friends, but they recede into the background. Everything does. Bile roils at the base of my gut. My knees shake. My teeth chatter against each other in my mouth.

I shiver uncontrollably, even though I'm not cold. I think *Did he see me?*

What do I do if he sees me?

What do I do if he doesn't?

Because I can't stand the not knowing, I eventually walk up to the bar, moving slowly because of the way it feels as if my legs might collapse beneath me. I slide onto a stool directly behind him where he waits for his turn at the dartboard. I incline my head toward the bartender. "Bud. Bottle," I say, and at the sound of my voice, he glances over his shoulder. He sees me staring down at my fingers folding creases into limp dollar bills. He smiles. Says, "Hey, what's up?" in a way so casual it shatters me.

I match his laid-back calm because, as a woman, I have already learned that a man's comfort is more important than my own. My body knows down to its bones and breath and blood that to put a man at ease is to protect itself. I smile and make nice because to acknowledge my pain doesn't make me strong. Making him see my pain—making him aware of his role in it—only makes me an antagonistic, hysterical bitch.

We make small talk. The kind of *how are yous* and *what're you up tos* that barely scratch the surface. When I make a joke about how some things never change, about how he is still picking up younger women in local bars (which is how we initially met), he is immediately defensive. "Really?" he says, shaking his head. "After all this time, you're *still* mad at me?"

He turns away, effectively dismissing me, making me relive all of the moments he ever dismissed what I was feeling, what I wanted, what I was or was not ready for. I'm not sure how to respond—because yes, I *am* angry, but no, I don't want to create a scene—so I take my beer and go. I am lightheaded as I make my way back to the end of the bar where the other karaoke singers are gathered, my cheeks on fire, my fingertips numb, my hands cold and damp. An old friend is doing a serviceable "Mack the Knife" and people are chatting and laughing as I drop down into a chair, my thumbs drawing whorls and zig-zags into the condensation on my beer bottle. I use a fingernail to scrape at the label, slowly coming back into myself even as my legs continue to shake.

It is then that I realize: *that man broke me, and I am still broken.*

Ten more years pass. Ten years in which I can't help but be aware of the fact that the person who left such an indelible mark on my life is seemingly oblivious to what he did to me. The entire course of my life shifted because of what occurred between us. Years of pain during intercourse. Useless medical tests that provided no answers. Disinterest in intimacy. *Fear* of intimacy.

I have a career in which I write about women's health, sexuality, assault, and consent. It is a career built upon a single evening—his shorts sliding down his legs, my thighs straining toward each other.

He is still shuffling from local bar to local bar, playing darts, drinking beer.

Please don't misunderstand. I feel strong now. For the most part, I've put anger behind me. As okay as I am, however, and as strong as I am, I am still not strong enough to use the word "rape." I still use words like "nonconsensual" and "coercive." After all these years, I still don't believe I can lay claim to that other label. I still don't entirely believe that I deserve to. I don't believe that my experience merits such a decisive, ugly word. I discredit my own experience, and all of the thoughts and feelings and sexual struggles that followed, because I know of so many other women who have had experiences that were exponentially worse. In the grand scheme of things, what Travis did to me was thoughtless and shitty. My reaction to it, however, has been unwarranted and overblown.

In 2015—a time when I was writing articles for members of a professional organization comprised of sexuality educators, counselors, and therapists—I learned about the many definitions of rape and sexual assault that exist.

At the time I was doing this research, issues of rape, sexual assault, and consent had been especially prominent in the public conversation. *Rolling Stone* magazine had published "A Rape on Campus," and then retracted it when many parts of the story were called into question. Jon Krakauer had published *Missoula*, a meticulously reported piece of narrative journalism on a series of sexual assaults at the University of Montana. Women had begun to come forward in order to accuse Bill Cosby of rape, and the media exploded. It was still two years before we would see the torrent of sexual assault allegations against Harvey Weinstein, Louis C.K., and so many other men in positions of power but, in the wake of these early pieces and others, it seemed everyone was suddenly talking about consent: what it meant, how it might be granted, and who was responsible for it.

A part of me felt a vicious glee. Men were finally being called out for the things they had done. The deplorability of their actions was finally being acknowledged on the national stage.

Quickly, however, this dialogue felt useless. A public conversation had begun, but it only seemed to amplify the hopelessness of those who had been victimized, the impossibility of them ever achieving justice. Instead of finding closure, women were being put on trial for the crimes that had been perpetrated upon them.

Why would one ever speak the word *rape* out loud? It's bad enough to spend years blaming oneself for one's own victimization. Why invite the rest of the world to do the same?

Meanwhile, in the course of my own research, I learned that 68 percent of sexual assaults are never reported to the police.[25] This didn't surprise me. I already knew that, in many cases, women are afraid to report. They blame themselves for what happened. They feel ashamed. They fear no one will believe them.

These reactions by those who have been sexually assaulted are not unreasonable. Among the media, the general public, and even law enforcement, there are often elaborate conspiracy theories built up and picked apart to explain away the reasons for women's allegations. There is victim blaming. Doubt and outrage. Concern over the assailant's very bright future. In the face of all this, is it so surprising that many women choose to remain silent?

It seems that even the concept of rape itself can be difficult to pin down. And issues of sexual assault and consent can be just as unwieldy. Or at least it can sometimes seem so to those who are struggling to define what they have experienced.

As I dug through more research, I learned that many male college students report that they have never

---

25 "National Crime Victimization Survey." Bureau of Justice Statistics (BJS). Accessed June 06, 2016. http://www.bjs.gov/index .cfm?ty=dcdetail.

committed rape, nor would they ever rape, declarations that come into question when we learn that these very same men are not actually aware that the sexually aggressive actions they would consider engaging in do, in fact, constitute rape.[26] For example, a majority of participants in one study said they would "coerce somebody to intercourse by holding them down." But they wouldn't consider this sexually aggressive behavior to constitute rape. Participants also admitted that if a woman said "no," to their sexual advances, they would consider it merely a token resistance commonly used among women. In short, no means no, except not all of the time. In fact, most of the time, *no* apparently means that a woman is just being coy. Meanwhile, 35 percent of sexual assault victims didn't report their assault because it was "unclear that it was a crime or that harm was intended."[27]

More recent research shows that a majority of men confuse sexual interest with consent.[28] Researchers hypothesize that this is because of infuriatingly persistent beliefs in rape myths ("When a woman says no, she

26 Sarah R. Edwards., Kathryn A. Bradshaw, and Verlin B. Hinsz. "Denying Rape but Endorsing Forceful Intercourse: Exploring Differences Among Responders." *Violence and Gender* 1, no. 4 (2014): 188–93. doi:10.1089/vio.2014.0022.

27 Christopher P. Krebs, Phd, Christine H. Lindquist, PhD, Tara D. Warner, M.A., Bonnie S. Fisher, PhD, and Sandra L. Martin, PhD "The Campus Sexual Assault (CSA) Study." National Criminal Justice Reference Service. December 2007. Accessed June 6, 2016. https://www.ncjrs.gov/pdffiles1/nij/grants/221153.pdf.

28 Ashton M. Lofgreen, Richard E. Mattson, Samantha A. Wagner, Edwin G. Ortiz, and Matthew D. Johnson. "Situational and Dispositional Determinants of College Men's Perception of Women's Sexual Desire and Consent to Sex: A Factorial Vignette Analysis." *Journal of Interpersonal Violence*, November 02, 2017. doi:10.1177/0886260517738777.

really means yes"), and the cultural conditioning that causes men to embrace the norms of hypermasculinity, male-stereotyped behavior that values physical strength, aggression, and sexuality. The researchers behind a 2017 study championed the creation of programs that would empower women to assertively state their sexual desires and that would teach men about the necessity for affirmative consent.

In reading these statistics, it is clearer to me that my once-boyfriend may not have realized that what he did was wrong. How could I blame him for his ignorance when our legal system can't even agree upon what rape is? When the definitions for rape and sexual assault differ from state to state and organization to organization? How could I blame this man who was raised in a society that teaches its young boys that they are entitled to women's bodies? How could I blame him when I myself didn't even know how to name what happened?

When boys snap our bra straps in junior high, we're told to laugh it off as an adorable sign that the boy in question likes us.

We're told, "Boys will be boys."

When a young man sexually assaults a young woman, he is given every benefit of the doubt. He didn't know what he was doing. He didn't realize she wasn't into it. He interpreted her clothes or her actions or her smile as an invitation.

He didn't realize.

Boys will be boys.

When I was researching all of the varying definitions for rape, sexual assault, and consent, I found myself on the website for the Rape, Abuse, and Incest National

Network (RAINN), where they had a page specifically for those men and women who were not sure whether or not they had been raped. Titled appropriately enough "Was I Raped?", the page suggested readers ask themselves three questions in the event they were unsure about an incident:

Were both of us old enough to consent to sexual activity according to state law?

Did either of us have an illness or disability that would adversely impact our ability to consent?

Did we both agree to take part?

Though I was working, I found myself reading these questions not as a journalist, but as someone who needed to know, for herself: *What happened to me? What should I call it? Does only one "no" out of three mean it doesn't count?*

Is my pain legitimate?

After these three initial questions, the page listed additional frequently asked questions for those who were still unsure. Which I was. So I continued reading. These bonus questions tackled seemingly gray areas such as those instances wherein one did not resist physically, or wherein the assailant was a romantic partner.

As I scanned through the questions, I made myself remember again. His shorts on the shag carpeting. My thighs.

But I didn't say no, said the voice in my head.

But I let it happen.

But I loved him.

This page has since been removed from the RAINN website, but there is a new page on the legal role of consent that goes into even greater depth on how consent is analyzed, and on what might impair one's capacity to consent.[29]

"Why didn't you fight back?" women are often asked, with the assumption that if they don't have the scars and the blood and the bruises to prove their resistance, the sex was consensual. Skeptics are more willing to believe a woman wanted it—and that she is only just now experiencing morning-after regret—than they are willing to understand the ways in which a body can protect itself from physical harm, the ways in which the brain can flick a switch in favor of self-preservation.

Back then, I didn't understand it myself. I didn't realize that my silence and inaction were a natural, behavioral response to threat. I didn't learn until many years later that the freeze response is a common response to sexual assault among women . . . and also one of the reasons women who come forward are so often discredited.

I thought that, because of my silence, what Travis did was excusable. After all, how could he know that he'd taken something I didn't intend to give? I was not explicit enough. I was not loud enough. I squeezed my thighs together. I said, "I'm not sure."

But "I'm not sure" is not the same as "no."

In New Jersey, where I was born and where I grew up and where I still live, aggravated sexual assault in the first degree is defined as "committing an act of sexual penetration with another person" under a set of possible circumstances, including the use of "physical force or

29 "Legal Role of Consent." RAINN. Accessed November 24, 2017. https://www.rainn.org/articles/legal-role-consent.

coercion," and with severe personal injury sustained by the victim.

"Severe personal injury" is further defined to mean "severe bodily injury, disfigurement, disease, incapacitating mental anguish or chronic pain."

In trying to determine whether or not an assault has occurred, however, who gets to diagnose your mental anguish as "incapacitating?" You or the courts? And how long does your pain have to linger before it is considered "chronic?" Did my pain count, even though it only emerged years later and then, eventually, disappeared?

After the retracted *Rolling Stone* article and the publication of Krakauer's *Missoula*, people finally began to turn their attention to the epidemic of sexual assault on college campuses. Among sexuality educators, college administrators, and even legislators, there was a strong push for the incorporation of consent education in high school sexuality education courses, and as part of college orientations. And not just consent, but "affirmative sexual consent." In a shift away from the long-held wisdom that "no means no"—a mindset that places the onus of sexually aggressive behavior on victims who are often too terrified or paralyzed to express their dissent—the definition of consent has evolved. Instead of "no means no," many have now taken up the chorus of "yes means yes," which means that explicit consent—a "yes" that cannot be mistaken for anything but enthusiastic agreement—must be given by both parties.

As we redefine consent, it becomes harder and harder to disregard the validity of my own feelings, and of the ways in which I've chosen to respond to this one incident in my life.

After all, I never said yes.

Still, that word—*rape*—remains so hard say, and I continue to be reluctant to apply it to my own experience.

Am I perpetuating the problem?

How can teach my daughter to speak her own truth if I still don't know how to speak my own?

10 | WHAT WILL I TEACH MY DAUGHTER?

I used to take my daughter to a weekly music class at a Presbyterian church around the corner. We'd all sit in a circle and clap our hands and dance with scarves and sing about owls and oak trees. Emily had always been slow to warm up around other people, so she mostly just sat in my lap until the hour had passed, at which point she would decide that *this moment* would be a fabulous time to run around in circles, shrieking with glee.

One week, as we were sitting and swaying to a lullaby, the boy next to Emily reached out and took her hand.

She pulled her hand away immediately, giving him the same look she gave me that time she tried eating cat food and realized she had just made a horrible life decision.

I tried not to snort too loudly. I was delighted to see Emily taking ownership of her own body and setting boundaries, even if it was only an unconsidered reflex.

When we're around other people, I try to make it clear that she does not have to hug or kiss anyone unless she wants to, even if her momentary rejection of someone's physical affection shatters their heart into a million pieces.

One time, as my parents left my house, my mom asked Emily if she could get a goodbye kiss.

"No!" said Emily, smiling smugly because toddlers are really good at looking smug.

"Can *I* get a goodbye kiss?" asked my dad.

Em walked over to him and leaned forward, pursing her lips.

"Thanks a *lot*, Emily!" said my mom, and Emily laughed. She didn't understand that these decisions were a rehearsal for what was still to come. She was just being a toddler.

It may seem drastic to equate the unwanted physical affections of loved ones with the unwanted physical advances that come later in life. And that's certainly not what I'm doing here. Rather, I'm trying to show my daughter that making these decisions about personal boundaries early on in life will help her internalize the knowledge that her body is hers and hers alone. I'm trying to teach her that the ability to say "no" is a muscle that must be flexed early on and often until it becomes hard. Until it becomes strong.

But how do I convey this importance to her? How do I tell her that being comfortable with saying "no" is imperative in a world in which "I don't know" or "I'm not sure" or absolute silence are taken as signs to keep going? How do I convey to her that, even when a woman doesn't say "no," it doesn't necessarily mean she's given consent? How do I make her understand that if a man takes what is not his to take, it is not her fault?

This education feels like a massive undertaking, and it is tempting to assume that these are lessons she will not need, that she will live a life that is easy and free from the mortifications every single woman experiences in one form or another.

I hope with all my heart that she is never in a situation in which a boy thinks it's okay to snap her bra just because he likes her. That a boy never calls her a slut just because he's pissed off and "slut" is the nastiest word he can think of to use. That she is never afraid walking home alone, never has to sprint the final block to her apartment because she is being followed. That she never has to figure out how to react when a man on the street tells her she has "nice tits." That she never feels guilty for telling a man he cannot come in when he follows her home, drunk, from the club. That she never feels she has to value a man's comfort over her own. That she never needs to ask herself: *Was that rape?*

But I know the statistics and I've heard the stories and, Jesus Christ, did you ever just scan through the #YesAllWomen or #MeToo hashtags on Twitter? Because yes. *All* women.

It terrifies me, but I know that just by being a girl, Emily is at risk for any number of dangerous or degrading situations through no fault of her own.

Margaret Atwood once wrote that "Men are afraid that women will laugh at them. Women are afraid that men will kill them."

I've stopped being afraid for myself.

Now I'm just afraid for my daughter.

* * *

When I began writing about sex in 2002, I wrote to fix myself. I reviewed Pocket Rockets and Rabbit Habits and wearable vibrators like the She Shell because I wanted to reclaim my sexual agency, to figure out what made me feel good. I reviewed cardio striptease classes and books like Carol Queen's *Exhibitionism for the Shy* because I wanted to be confident. I researched female sexual dysfunction because I felt defective. Those sex parties? They allowed me—for just one night—to feel as if I were someone else. Someone better. Someone whole.

My very first print magazine clip in *Playgirl* was a travel piece on sex parties around the world. My article was illustrated with a drawing of a massive orgy. Despite the explicitness of both the content and the artwork, my mother was so proud of me she made photocopies and carried them around in her purse so she could show my story to friends and coworkers.

Still, I know she believed this sex writing thing was just a phase. She didn't realize that toy and porn reviews would soon be followed by service pieces and advice columns and personal essays and, eventually, collaborations with sexuality professionals. She didn't know this would become the thing that defined me, the thing I am, a professional writer who built her life around the search for sexual reclamation.

Fifteen years after first starting down this path, I realized I wasn't broken.

Once I had that epiphany, I thought maybe I was done.

By that time, I was burnt out on writing the same old listicles about orgasms and libido. A job working with sexologists would soon reignite my passion for writing about female sexuality but, in that moment, I felt as if I had come to the end of a very long quest—a quest in which the thing I had been searching for was not at all what I had expected.

Is this all I needed? I asked myself.

Does this mean I'm done?

I spent a year floating. Looking for a reason to write. Looking for something to work toward. At the end of that year, I was given the opportunity to work for AASECT, a professional organization for sexuality professionals dedicated to furthering the idea that sexuality and sexual health are an integral part of overall health and well-being. I took the job despite worrying that I was getting in over my head. A month later, I learned I was pregnant.

By the time this book comes out, the realization that there is nothing wrong with my libido, or with my body, will be even further in my past. My daughter's fourth birthday will have come and gone. I'll be thirty-eight, and my life will presumably be perfect. After all, I will have all the answers I spent years searching for. I'll have the child I always dreamed of. And I'll be a published author, something I've wanted for as long as I've wanted to be a mother. There will be nothing left to achieve, right? At that point, I'll be able to ride off into the sunset with my adorable family and my perfectly adequate sex life and perhaps even a box of books to hand-sell to unwitting bystanders.

Here. Hold a copy of my book while I laugh so hard I eventually devolve into sobbing.

Don't get me wrong. For the first time in my life, I feel as if I finally have my shit together. For the most part. But I've found—again and again—that when you accomplish one huge thing on your massive life to-do list, new things emerge.

When Emily was born, it felt as if my heart had grown so many sizes that my breastbone was shattered, my ribs exploded outward, my body one large, exposed nerve overwhelmed by sensations of love and fear. After Michael's two-week paternity leave, and another week with my mom, I was left alone with Emily. Two months into new motherhood, I started working again, using my foot to lull Em to sleep in her Rock 'n Play as I conducted phone interviews, breastfeeding Em while I typed up articles, running back and forth between my computer and the changing pad and my pumping bra, casting frantic glances at the rest of the house, which slowly descended into a messy ruin. Where before I had been practicing yoga four to six times a week and meditating once or twice a day (a crucial mood stabilizer now that I no longer took antidepressants), I was now barely practicing at all. It took only a few weeks of this juggling act before I found myself crying off and on during the day, holding Em close so she couldn't see my tears.

Still, I continued trying to do it all, unwilling to pay for childcare, unwilling to stop working, even though there really wasn't much left of me to devote to my marriage, or to myself. I had been through this muck before, after all—the muck of anxiety and depression that seemed to perpetually weigh me down and to weigh on my marriage. The only difference was that my fights with Michael had evolved from whether we would sleep together to who would purée the apples. Living with depression had always made it hard to look forward, to even know what I was working toward. Despite my inability to look toward the future, however, there was one thing I knew with absolute certainty: I did not want a second child. Hell, I was barely holding it together with one.

The problem was that over ten years ago, I wanted something different. When we first discussed our future together—beautiful home, five thousand cats (well, one of those was still up for discussion)—we agreed that we both wanted two children. And Michael still wanted that. But having Emily forced me to shift my life in so many ways. Without my yoga practice, I felt unhealthy, both physically and mentally. I stopped teaching yoga, too, which was previously a source of great fulfillment. And I was forced to pull back from my writing and editing work since everything I *did* tackle took at least twice as long to accomplish. As a woman who wanted to be defined by more than her role as a mother, I wasn't willing to cede any more ground.

On top of that, I was absolutely in love with my child. So much so that everything I was learning over the course of my time with AASECT—and everything I'd ever learned through my other journalistic work— left me paralyzed with fear. The research I did on sexuality education and sexual violence and various forms of gender bias only served to keep at the forefront of my mind all of the ways in which my daughter would be unsafe as she grew into womanhood. How could I possibly protect my daughter, have a successful career, continue to love my husband, and maintain my sanity with the added pressure of a second child?

The plan had always been for Michael to get a vasectomy after we had a second child. It's a plan we both agreed to. But after having Emily, I found I didn't want the same things anymore. I asked Michael to get the procedure done immediately. He refused.

It didn't help that everyone and their mother (including my own mother) was asking us when we planned to have a second child. For a long time, I simply laughed off their comments with a smile that was more like a grimace because it felt selfish and hypocritical of me to discuss my wants and my fears when, for three and a half years, I'd wanted a child so desperately. After a while, though, even that small bit of playacting became too hard.

Marriage is a partnership, but I can't help but feel that when it comes to having children, a woman's wants should be more heavily weighted. I still remember the bloodwork and the other tests I had to undergo when we enlisted the help of fertility doctors: the daily injections, the early morning ultrasounds, the constant monitoring, the assumption that my body was the problem. I remember the eventual pregnancy, fairly easy, but not without its own helping of 24/7 nausea, cankles, and nighttime back pain. I remember the labor, the contractions, the vomiting, the pushing, the glut of blood that poured out from between my legs, the adult diapers I wore for weeks afterward. I can feel my vagina wincing every time I imagine what it might be like to do it all over again.

After the birth, when I went in for a follow-up

appointment with my obstetrician, she prescribed me a new birth control pill. Later on, because Michael still wouldn't consider a vasectomy, I had an IUD inserted into my uterus. After that, I relished telling people that I had my uterus on lockdown. "NOPE," I'd respond when asked if I planned to have a second. "I had an IUD stuck up into my hoo-ha," I'd say, using hand gestures and everything.

Still, after about a year with my IUD, I began to notice an unpleasant—and strong—smell wafting from my nether regions. It became a new and demoralizing source of shame. I suspected bacterial vaginosis, an infection that can become more likely when you have an IUD, but the test came back negative. Still, by then, my patience had just about run out. I was sick of being the only one to take responsibility for family planning, and I was annoyed that Michael seemed to be biding his time, waiting for me to change my mind about having a second child. My vaginal issues had also introduced a sliver of doubt as to the efficacy of my IUD and, every time we had sex, I was terrified I would be among the tiny percentage of women for whom an IUD had failed (0.8%[30]). And I knew that, even though I was 100 percent certain about not wanting another child, if I had an unplanned pregnancy, I would keep it.

Again, this conundrum of mine is nothing new. Not for women. There have always been far fewer contraceptive options for men and, as a result, it has long been assumed that pregnancy prevention is the responsibility

30 "Contraception." February 9, 2017. https://www.cdc.gov /reproductivehealth/contraception/index.htm.

of women. Perhaps because of this, research on new contraceptive methods for men has been limited. Every so often, we see stories about mildly horrifying "break-throughs" that are still in the testing phases, but not far enough along to enter U.S. clinical trials. These have included progestin and polymer gel injections, testosterone implants, and more.[31] None of these bright and shining possibilities ever seems to come to fruition, however, and so women . . . just take care of it.

New research shows that, in addition to shouldering most of the physical burden of preventing pregnancy, women shoulder most of the mental and emotional labor, too.[32] Well, duh. What this means is that this imbalance is about more than just the invasiveness of an implant or an intrauterine device. It's about more than the chemicals we are forced to put into our bodies. On top of all that, it's also about the time and mental space we have to give to finding a gynecologist we trust. Determining the right contraceptive option for us. Seeing if it takes, or whether or not there are adverse side effects we might not be able to live with. And in the case of options such as the pill or the sponge or the cervical cap, using it consistently. Because if we screw up any of this, failure rates skyrocket. And if things go sideways, it's our asses on the line. And later on, of course, if we keep that unplanned

31 Samantha Allen. "Seriously, Though: Why Hasn't Male Birth Control Happened Yet?" Splinter. November 29, 2016. https://splinternews.com/seriously-though-why-hasn-t-male-birth-control-happen-1793863988.

32 Katrina Kimport. "More Than a Physical Burden: Women's Mental and Emotional Work in Preventing Pregnancy." *The Journal of Sex Research*, April 18, 2017, 1-10. doi:10.1080/00224499.2017.1311834.

pregnancy, women are also more often shunted into the role of primary caregiver. Is it too much to ask that I have final say on whether or not I take on all of that again?

Explaining all of this to Michael—convincing him that having an only child really is the best option for the both of us ("Emily is superior to all other children! How could we possibly build upon perfection?")—has been a long game. And it's been yet another stressor on our sex life. But did I *really* think that our intimate life would magically become perfect just because I'd learned that our struggles in bed weren't a "me problem" but an "us problem?"

In the meantime, however, and despite some hiccups, our marriage feels stronger than it ever has before. Though studies show that marital satisfaction declines after having children because of shifts in focus and responsibility and identity,[33] that has not been our personal experience. Even with arguments about division of labor, and parenting-related exhaustion, and the occasional dirty dishes-induced meltdown, we're rocking it. When I ask Michael why he thinks we're so rock solid these days despite the stresses of parenthood, he makes a good point. "We're living the life we wanted to live," he says, referring to our protracted attempts to start a family, "and we don't take it for granted. We love being parents and seeing ourselves in her and sharing the world with her."

---

33 Brian D. Doss, Galena K. Rhoades, Scott M. Stanley, and Howard J. Markman. "The effect of the transition to parenthood on relationship quality: An 8-year prospective study." *Journal of Personality and Social Psychology 96*, no. 3 (March 2009): 601–19. doi:10.1037/a0013969.

He pauses.

"Wait, why does it feel like you're interviewing me right now?"

Such is life when you're married to a writer.

As much as I love sharing the world with Em, I still wrestle with how much I should shield her from, despite knowing that every dark part of the world will reveal itself to her eventually. How can I control the unconscious forms of gender bias she is exposed to on a daily basis from her grandparents, at her preschool, and even from strangers? How do I explain to relatives that we don't force her to give hugs and kisses—though we do encourage polite hellos and goodbyes? When I try, they look at me as if I'm crazy, or as if I have berated them for their attempts at showing affection. It feels impossible to push back against years upon years of cultural conditioning.

Even those who should have absolutely zero say in my parenting choices think I'm a nut job. When I took this very chapter of my book to a local writing critique group, reading aloud the section about the fears I held for my daughter, the man next to me drew his brows together and pursed his lips, troubled. "I have a niece who just turned eighteen," he said, "and none of these things you worry about have ever crossed my mind." He tapped his pencil against the table. Looked up at me. "I think . . ." he said, critiquing my life instead of my writing, "that maybe you're making things too complicated."

Here. Hold my fourth coffee of the day while I punch something.

It's tough to raise a daughter with this additional

layer of awareness when it seems as if the rest of the world is content to stick to the same old gender binary-bound lessons. I suppose that this—like every other aspect of motherhood—is something I have to figure out as I go along. Luckily, the knowledge I've amassed over the years—and especially the recent knowledge about sex ed techniques—puts me at an advantage.

My daughter is now at that age where her legs dangle over the edge of her changing pad, and where every errant flip or flail of her chubby thighs can knock over tubes of diaper rash cream and body lotion or send her hurtling off the table and onto the hardwood floor.

So I distract her by quizzing her.

"Where's your head?" I ask as I undo her diaper and wipe her down, and she brings both hands to her head.

"Good job! Where's your stomach?" I ask as I put a new diaper in place, and she taps her belly.

"Yup! Where are your toes?" I ask as I bring the diaper flaps across her belly and Velcro the whole shebang shut. She extends her legs and looks at her toes. "Wee wee wee?" she asks, because that is what she calls them ever since she learned "This little piggie."

"Yes!" I say, pretending to eat her toes. "And where is your vulva?" I ask.

She does a Michael Jackson crotch grab.

"Yes!" I say. "Yay!" I say. I wrestle her jeans up to her waist and wrestle her feet through the leg holes as she smiles and claps her hands.

"Yay!" she says and claps her hands together. "Vulva," she says, and it is the most adorable thing ever.

In my two years working with AASECT, I learned so

much about sexuality, information I couldn't learn from sex toy test drives and sex parties alone. I grilled sexuality educators in particular for information on how to raise a sexually healthy child from birth on, on how to impart the sex-positive values that would best serve them as they grew older. This—teaching her the proper names for her body parts—is easy.

But I know that being my daughter's educator will only become harder. That the lessons will become more complicated.

I am only just now starting to consider how I might best teach her about gender and privacy and body agency. What will I do when she someday walks in on me and Michael having sex? What will I say when she starts asking questions about masturbation or sexual decision making? How will I handle those warring needs to have a daughter who is sexually autonomous and confident, and to have a daughter who is safe?

What will I teach my daughter?

I start with the small stuff. With her body parts. With teaching her how to be someone who loves her own body.

I remember being eleven and being shamed for never having shaved my legs. I remember being twelve and wishing my body invisible. I remember Travis showing me—when I was only nineteen—that my body was not my own. Not really. I spent the majority of my life feeling great ambivalence for my body.

But then, when I was thirty-three, my belly grew large with the baby inside of me and I found that I didn't mind. Later that year, I give birth to a baby girl, my legs spread wide, my vulva on display, so much blood spilling out of me that my OB/GYN went pale, and I was not ashamed. Emily soon became an extension of my body, her tiny fingers splayed across my breast, her lips on my nipple. As she grew older and stopped nursing, my body remained hers. I found that I didn't mind. Let her have my body, I thought, if only to learn more about her own.

She now follows me into the bathroom, sometimes even pulling her stool between my legs and leaning her elbows on my thighs. "Mommy going pee pee?" she asks. "Yes," I say, and I explain to her the steps for using the potty. Other times, we play peekaboo while I shower, my hair piled atop my head with soap suds. In the evenings, I change into my pajamas in front of her.

She pats my thighs. "Oh!" she says, alarmed, which makes me laugh.

She points to my chest. "Is that a bra? Is that a bra?"

"Yes, sweetheart. That's a bra."

We lay on the bed together and she pulls up the bottom hem of my pajama top and pats my belly, places a finger in my belly button. We each pat our own bellies, playing what we refer to as the "tum drum."

There are periods of time in which I revel in my body's strength and flexibility, in which I feel healthy and comfortable with who I am. In those moments, it is easy to teach my daughter how to love her own body.

But then there are periods in which I stand before the mirror and my gaze goes immediately to my "thunder thighs," to the pooch that slops over my waistband, to the vast expanse of me that seems to fill the entire full-length mirror. At these times, it is a struggle to not use words like "fat" or "muffin top" or "jiggly" or "ugly."

But I don't want to use those words in front of my daughter. I don't want her to internalize their message, though I know she'll be exposed to them eventually, somewhere.

Even when I am hating my own body, I still make sure to tell her how beautiful she is.

I tell her that she is perfect.

But I am not the perfect mother.

One day, as I was dumping my bedroom garbage into the larger kitchen garbage can, a mess of crumpled-up tissues and string cheese wrappers and clothing tags spilled out onto the floor.

"Fuuuuuuuuuuuuuck," I bellowed, momentarily forgetting my young daughter—who now absorbs every single word and phrase that slips past my lips—standing beside me.

"Fuuuuuuuuuuuuuuuug!" she repeated, beaming up at me, a sippy cup of milk clutched in her hands, milk dripping down her chin.

My gaze snapped to Michael's. "Don't react," he mouthed at me, and I pressed my lips together and sucked in my cheeks to prevent myself from spluttering out laughter.

Still. In the grand scheme of things, I think learning a curse word or five isn't all that terrible. I'd rather she learn "fuck" or "goddammit" as a result of my careless-ness than learn that her words and emotions are some-thing to be suppressed. I'd rather her start saying "Jesus Christ!" than learn that her thighs are worth scrutiny, or that the way others perceive her is a measure of her worth, or that the attentions of men are her responsibility. I imagine she'll pick up a lot of interesting vocabulary as a result of the work that I do or carry a lot of knowledge that others her age might not have access to. Other parents may wish she'd keep that knowledge to herself. But young girls know—just as I know—that knowledge is power.

My two-year-old daughter sat on my lap, attempting to rip open an eight-inch-long canister of forty condoms. This massive combo pack—plus three other packs and a folder filled with promotional materials—had been sent to me by a condom manufacturer I was referencing in an article about innovations in condom design.

"Want open?" my daughter asked, her fingernails scrabbling against the plastic edges.

And because I didn't think it was necessary for her to know what a condom was quite yet, I tried to convince her that the tube of lubricated latex prophylactics was actually a giant maraca.

"Shake it like this. See?" I jiggled it up and down so that each individually wrapped condom bumped up against the side of the container with a muffled clatter.

She remained unconvinced.

"Want open?"

I am only just now coming to terms with the fact that if something is accessible, Emily will access it. She went through a phase where she pulled garbage out of the garbage can. One time, I found her playing in the litter box as if it were a sandbox, using the poop scoop like a shovel. She has snatched tubs of lip balm and tubes of hand cream from my nightstand, opening them up and sometimes ingesting their contents. She has wandered around with my giant bottle of lube or my copy of *Sex Object* or the review unit of a just-released vibrator.

"Our daughter is wandering around with a vibrator," Michael once shouted as I was in the bathroom, face bent close to the mirror, flossing my teeth.

"Is she?" I shouted back.

Eventually, after I finished what I was doing, I took it from her, gently, careful not to freak out over the fact that she was handling an object designed to stimulate the clitoris. "This belongs to mommy," I said. "Why don't you not play with the things that belong to mommy?"

And then I briefly considered buying a steel safe with a combination lock for all of my adult toys and accessories.

As someone who writes about women's health and sexuality for a living, I feel an enormous pressure to raise my daughter in a sex-positive household. I want her to learn that her body and her sexuality are not cause for shame. That masturbation is a perfectly acceptable way to explore her body, and to learn about what feels good. I want her to grow up with enough knowledge to make smart, healthy decisions. I want her to be able to protect herself because I know that I cannot rely upon other parents, school administrators, and teachers to teach boys that a girl's body is not theirs to take.

There is so much to teach her, and I am scared that I will forget something important. Raising a daughter feels so much more terrifying than raising a son.

It took me fifteen years to feel satisfied with who I am sexually. I don't want it to take that long for my daughter. I want it to be something she *is* from the very beginning.

These days, there are fewer sex toys showing up on my doorstep in their "discreet" packaging, ambiguous names like "Pagnucci Development Group Inc." listed under the return address. After all, there's not much more for me to learn from the latest and greatest ergonomically designed vibrator. How much positive change can I possibly effect from writing up yet another piece on sex toy technology?

Instead, I spend far more time interviewing sexuality educators and volunteering my time to my local Planned Parenthood affiliate. Knowing as much as I do about the state of sex education, I feel as if I have no choice but to be an advocate for improved sex ed in whatever way I can. I know that I cannot take anything for granted. I know that I cannot trust that my daughter will get the information she needs from anyone but me.

How do you teach someone how to be a woman? What does that even mean?

I write in order to figure that out. Instead of writing to fix myself, I write to fix her future.

11 | THE THINGS WE MUST DO

He grabbed me from behind, his arms so skinny and his grip so tight I could feel his bones digging into my skin. My upper arms were pinned tight to my body, and I knew they'd be bruised later. I didn't think I'd be able to get enough leverage, but I acted anyway. I strained my arms forward while I simultaneously heaved my butt back. I got him right in the solar plexus and he groaned, stumbling back a few steps. I was free.

"That was pretty good," said Michael.

"Yeah, I didn't think it was gonna work," I admitted.

"Well, it worked," he said.

"The powers of the butt!" I crowed. I did a triumphant fist pump.

For the past few weeks, I'd been taking self-defense classes for women and gender-nonconforming folks at an anti-violence education center in Brooklyn, practicing the moves at home so my body could begin to internalize them. For years, I'd been doing research on female sexual dysfunction, on rape culture, on the general co-opting of female sexuality by our culture at large. But I felt fatigued by my focus on everything that was wrong. I wanted to learn more about the women who had moved past traumatic events, who were healing, who were doing what they could to reclaim their sexuality for themselves, and who were helping others do the same.

And so, I sought out sexuality educators who were spreading the gospel of "yes means yes." I spoke to app developers who were creating smartphone resources and alternative forms of sex ed for a new media generation. I contributed to an Indiegogo campaign for a safety device that would allow me to walk the streets alone feeling just a little bit more protected. And I took classes that allowed me to reconnect with my body. To be aware of its signals. To trust it.

I had wanted to take a self-defense class since my twenties, but I'd been scared. Going in, I was especially nervous that my lack of coordination would embarrass me within the very first hour of class. I mean, when I was thirteen, I was the only person on my basketball team to distinguish myself by never making a shot. In junior high, the only time I successfully blocked a soccer ball in gym class was accidental (I wasn't paying attention; the ball bounced off my thigh and clear across the field). I even sucked at bowling because of the lack of power in my swing. The ball would roll so slowly down the lane that, even when it hit directly in the pocket between the one and the three, I barely knocked over any pins.

I'd never done well at anything requiring physical strength, endurance, or agility. I didn't expect to perform adequately at *any* aspect of self-defense.

But surprisingly, the defensive moves came easy. I could demonstrate the blocks. I had perfect form when I air-kicked pretend shins, knees, and groins. I could list out all of the primary targets on an attacker's body—such as the nose and throat—followed by secondary targets like the feet and the solar plexus. And even though it grossed me out, I could easily remember *all* of the ways in which to poke, scratch, peck, or gouge out an attacker's eyes.

What I struggled with were the role-playing exercises. Particularly the role-playing exercises in which we were forced to set boundaries with someone we knew.

"You all deserve to have your boundaries respected," the instructors told us our very first week. We sat in a circle, discussing the reasons we might have for indulging someone who made us uncomfortable instead of assertively telling them to step off. It wasn't exactly a revelatory statement. Of *course* we deserved to have our boundaries respected.

But why was it so hard to set them in the first place?

During the sexual assault trial of former CBC host Jian Ghomeshi, when the complainant was asked why she'd stayed in Ghomeshi's home for an hour after he allegedly slapped and choked her, she said, "I didn't want to seem frosty and I didn't want to seem mad." Though many pointed to her behavior as a means of questioning the validity of her allegations, her statement is evidence of the "politeness conditioning"[34] all

34 Zosia Bielski. "How politeness conditioning can lead to confusion about sexual assaults." *The Globe and Mail*, March 20, 2016.

women experience.[35] It is an example of how women have been socially conditioned[36] to always be polite. To value another's comfort over their own.

Layered on top of this is the sense of safety that comes with remaining agreeable. With remaining compliant. After all, with confrontation comes the threat of retaliation.[37] Writer Hanna Brooks Olsen tackled the same topic in a piece titled—appropriately enough—"Why We Smile at Men Who Sexually Harass Us."[38] "The truth is, we don't have the luxury to ignore harassment," writes Olsen. "We engage, we're kind, because that is what keeps us safe."

This instinct is embedded in me, too. In the way I responded to the guy who took my hand and told me that hearing about my work made him horny. In my emotional reaction to the employer who used sexually explicit language with me on the regular.

One time, when walking through New York City on my way to speak on a panel about career diversification,

35 Elizabeth H. Dodd, Traci A. Giuliano, Jori M. Boutell, and Brooke E. Moran. "Respected or Rejected: Perceptions of Women Who Confront Sexist Remarks." *Sex Roles* 45, no. 7–8 (October 2001): 567–77.

36 Janet K. Swim and Laurie L. Hyers. "Excuse Me—What Did You Just Say?!: Women's Public and Private Responses to Sexist Remarks." *Journal of Experimental Social Psychology* 35, no. 1 (1999): 68–88. doi:10.1006/jesp.1998.1370.

37 Kristina A. Dickmann, Sheli D. Sillito Walker, Adam D. Galinsky, and Ann E. Tenbrunsel. "Double Victimization in the Workplace: Why Observers Condemn Passive Victims of Sexual Harassment." *Organization Science* 24, no. 2 (March & April 2013): 614–28. doi:10.1287/orsc.1120.0753.

38 Hanna Brooks Olsen. "Why Women Smile at Men Who Sexually Harass Us." Medium. February 23, 2016. Accessed August 02, 2017. https://medium.com/@mshannabrooks/why-women-smile-at -men-who-sexually-harass-us-cf4eeb90ed30.

I caught the eye of a man approaching from the opposite direction. He grinned at me and, reflexively, I responded with a smile of my own. As the corners of my mouth inched up, as my cheeks stretched into that smile, his lips moved.

"Nice tits," he said.

My smile melted.

The moment sticks with me because of how ashamed I felt.

Not angry.

Ashamed.

I felt ashamed for smiling back at him. I felt ashamed for encouraging him. I felt ashamed for being a woman with breasts.

But what else could I do? It was instinct.

Now, in a five-week self-defense class offered for free to those who had previously been victims of domestic violence and/or sexual assault, I was learning what else I could do. I was learning how to use my voice and my body language but, because of how I had been raised and the defensive mechanisms I had developed over the years, none of it was coming easy.

"Come on, Steph. Just one drink," a fellow classmate slurred at me, leaning in close, draping herself across my shoulders.

"Hey," I said, stepping back, raising a hand. "Not too close. Not too close." But she kept on coming. And I didn't know how to shut her down. I was afraid—even though we were only role-playing—that if I was firm, things would only be awkward later. I couldn't quite find that line between being assertive and what could possibly be seen as overreacting.

"It's hard, but I promise you: it *will* get easier," said one of the instructors.

I wasn't so sure. But this was why a class like this felt so necessary. Not just a self-defense class. An *empowerment* self-defense class.

When I first learned about empowerment self-defense (ESD), James W. Hopper, PhD, a clinical psychologist who advises and trains a variety of professionals on the neurobiology of trauma, had been chatting with me about our automatic response to danger. He mentioned that we can expect to change those automatic responses if we train ourselves in alternative methods to the extent that those new methods become instinctual.

"Nobody understands this better than the military," said Hopper. "All these drills they do before they're sent into battle. Things become habit. Then, when the bullets are flying, and people are dying, and they can't think straight, there are those habits to fall back on. What habits do most women have to fall back on? Nice girl habits. Like how to politely resist a guy who's trying to go further than she wants without hurting his feelings or angering him. These are the habits girls and women learn, and they're useless in a sexual assault. But the conditioning from an intensive self-defense course can overcome that."

He mentioned research he'd read on ESD courses,[39] self-defense that went beyond physical defensive techniques. These courses delved into gender conditioning

---

39 Jocelyn A Hollander. "Does Self-Defense Training Prevent Sexual Violence Against Women?" *Violence Against Women* 20, no. 3 (March 12, 2014): 252–69. doi:10.1177/1077801214526046.

and empowered girls and women to recognize the tendencies they had to react passively and politely. They helped women to develop new, more assertive habits.

I was intrigued. While a common critique of self-defense classes for women is that they place the onus of preventing sexual assault on the victim versus the perpetrator, I was tired of feeling powerless.

Lynne Marie Wanamaker, Deputy Director of the domestic violence organization Safe Passage, and an ESD instructor, calls this the self-defense paradox. On the one hand, she explains, there is only one person responsible for an assault: the perpetrator.

On the other hand, we can all work toward creating a safer world. There are things we can all do to increase our own safety.

Both are true.

"This is something we can never lose sight of," says Wanamaker. "It is not my fault that sexual violence exists in the world. I am never going to be responsible for that, no matter what. At the same time, there are things I can do to improve my situation. That's agency. That's empowerment. Our choices are limited because of oppression, but we always have choices and strengths we can bring to bear on our situation."

These are the truths ESD courses are built around. And so, courses are designed[40] to develop students'

---

40 Charlene Y. Senn, PhD, Misha Eliasziw, PhD, Paula C. Barata, PhD, Wilfreda E. Thurston, Ph.D., Ian R. Newby-Clark, PhD, H. Lorraine Radtke, PhD, and Karen L. Hobden, PhD "Efficacy of a Sexual Assault Resistance Program for University Women." *New England Journal of Medicine* 373, no. 14 (June 11, 2015): 1375 –376. doi:10.1056/nejmc1509345.

strengths, and to give them more choices. In order to achieve this, ESD schools offer more hours of programming, often providing self-defense series that are at least five weeks long. In addition to teaching physical self-defensive moves, there are also a greater number of interactive and practice exercises, including role-playing, group discussions, and partner work, with an emphasis on internalizing the options that will be most likely to remove you from danger.

"Women are trained to be desensitized to their own instincts," says Wanamaker. "We don't set boundaries over how we want to be treated and what's acceptable. Empowerment self-defense gives students the skills to set those boundaries, and to separate themselves from situations that don't feel okay to them. It allows them to overcome that initial instinct of not wanting to make a scene or hurt his feelings. It gets them past that emotional barrier, where they wonder 'Am I reading this right?' It enables them to notice what it feels like in their body when they feel unsafe or uncomfortable, to regulate that, and to come up with an intentional response."

Wanamaker also describes an environment in which everything is opt-in. "We practice the world we want to live in," she says. "If someone is uncomfortable, if they'd rather watch, that's fine, we normalize that, as opposed to other martial arts classes I've been in, where it's like, 'Come on! Aren't you here to get tough?' You can't underestimate what that feels like to practice that and have that normalized. That when I say 'no,' things stop. As a survivor, that never gets old for me. It continues to be magic for me, and I've been teaching since 1991."

Wanamaker mentions that she has a daughter, and I can't help asking her how she's brought some of those ESD lessons home. After all, it makes me think of my own daughter, and of how I struggle to teach her what I know, when appropriate. To raise her to be an empowered woman despite the urge to enfold her in the protective circle of my arms and never let go.

"My daughter's emotional self-awareness just dazzles me," says Wanamaker. "She really feels a right to what she feels. When she was four, she went a whole year with no kisses, and it was developmentally appropriate for her to assert that boundary. Every time I respected that boundary, I was creating that as the norm for her."

Wanamaker is insistent again on the importance of these lessons. "We don't say, 'This isn't your fault . . . wait for him to fix it,'" says Wanamaker. "I'll be damned if I'm going to sit here and wait for rape culture to end on its own."

Before leaving my self-defense class every night, I pinned my Athena device to the neck of my tank top, right below my clavicle, where it wouldn't draw the attention of others, but where I could reach for it easily without fumbling.

The device was sleek and circular with a black, elastomer front, the guts of it housed in a lightweight aluminum, rose gold-embellished casing. It was held fast to my top with a black, magnetic clasp. It featured a contoured design intended to guide my finger to the slightly recessed button, which—when pressed—would alert others to the fact that I was in danger.

If I tapped it twice, I could check in with my contacts,

letting them know where I was, and that I was okay. If I pressed it once, holding the button down, it would emit a loud beeping sound, drawing the attention of anyone in the vicinity and also sending a message to my emergency contacts, giving them the option to call me, call 911, find out my location, or request a check-in from me. If I tapped it quickly, three times, it would alert my contacts without making a sound. I could use this option if I was worried that the alarm might escalate the situation and put me in even more danger.

Securing the device to my top, I wondered if I would even have the wherewithal to go for it if I was ever in real danger. Or if I would feel silly pressing the button to check in with my emergency contacts if I felt merely uneasy. I'd been learning how to pay attention to where fear manifested in the body and how it felt, how to listen to my instincts. But women are used to being told that they're irrational[41] and overreactive and, as a result, I'd always doubted my own instincts.

Still, when I first stumbled upon the Indiegogo campaign for the Athena, I was excited. The thought of owning a discreet safety device was intriguing, and it seemed like a project that was worth supporting. So I did, giving enough money to ensure that I would receive my own device once they finished production. About a year and a half later, I received my device in the mail and literally squeed. Not only was I pleased to have a product intended to make me feel safer as a woman

41 Cecilia Tasca, Mariengela Rapetti, Mauro Giovanni Carta, and Bianca Fadda. "Women And Hysteria In The History Of Mental Health." *Clinical Practice & Epidemiology in Mental Health* 8 (October 19, 2012): 110–19. doi:10.2174/1745017901208010110.

out in the world, but I felt gratified knowing that I was supporting a company with an ambitious mission I could get behind.

The idea for the device itself was planted when Yasmine Mustafa spent six months trekking alone across South America. When she told her friends about the trip, they thought it sounded awesome, but they also worried it was dangerous. Mustafa went ahead and took the trip anyway, traveling across six different countries. She enjoyed her trip, but also found it distressing. During her travels, she met many women who shared with her their stories of assault.

Shortly after she returned home to Philadelphia, a brutal rape occurred just blocks from Mustafa's apartment. After this incident, she realized she had to shift course and do *something* in the face of all of this sexualized violence. Previously, this refugee from Kuwait had worked her way up through impossible odds, founding a company that developed affiliate marketing software for bloggers and even forming a Philadelphia chapter of Girl Develop It, teaching women how to code in an effort to close the gender gap in the tech field. Now, she wanted to use her tech and marketing know-how to get to the root of sexual violence. She formed ROAR for Good, the organization behind the Athena device.

In developing the device, Mustafa and her team wanted to create something different from what was already out there. In the case of weapons and pepper sprays, they worried that a user could possibly be overpowered and have their own device used against them. They wanted to create something that would deter attack without causing harm, and also allow users to get immediate help. And they wanted it to be readily available in the midst of an altercation.

Now, they have a ninety-nine-dollar device that, when paired with the free phone app, allows users to set up an emergency contacts list and compose pre-written alert messages that get sent out at the touch of a button. The app also aggregates relevant content, some of it intended to inspire, some of it intended to educate, and there is a rich resource component where those who have been victims of sexual assault, domestic violence, or harassment can find support. For example, one piece links out to a comic intended to help parents teach their kids about consent. Another piece references a RAINN resource about staying safe on campus. And yet another refers to a hashtag campaign about media representation.

The organization's next step is to develop a lower-cost version of the Athena for women in underdeveloped socioeconomic environments. After all, those who come from marginalized and lower-income populations tend to be at higher risk of assault and intimate partner violence (IPV). For example, women between the ages of twenty-five and twenty-nine with fewer than three years of college under their belt are more than twice as likely to have been raped than women in the same age group who had attended four or more years of college,[42] while young people who are not enrolled in college have

---

42 William George Axinn, Maura Elaine Bardos, and Brady Thomas West. "General population estimates of the association between college experience and the odds of forced intercourse." *Social Science Research*, October 31, 2017. doi:10.1016/j.ssresearch.2017.10.006.

a higher chance of experiencing sexual assault.[43] Meanwhile, women in the lowest income categories experience IPV at more than six times the rate of those in the highest income category.[44] African American women experience IPV at a much higher rate than their white counterparts,[45] American-Indian women are victimized at a rate more than double that of women of other races,[46] and the list goes on.[47] The statistics aren't much better for sexual minorities. Twenty-one percent of TGQN (transgender, genderqueer, nonconforming) college students have been sexually assaulted, compared to 18 percent of non-TGQN females, and 4 percent of non-TGQN males.[48] So when it comes to those who need protection the most, high-cost solutions are often not as feasible.

On top of greater accessibility for all, Anthony Gold, cofounder and the COO of ROAR for Good, says that

43 Sinozich, Sofi, and Lynn Langton, Ph.D. "Rape and Sexual Assault Victimization Among College-Age." *Bureau of Justice Statistics*. December 2014. Accessed December 12, 2017.

44 Erika Harrell, PhD, Lynn Langton, PhD, Marcus Berzofsky, DrPH, Lance Couzens, and Hope Smiley-McDonald, PhD "Household Poverty and Nonfatal Violent Victimization, *Bureau of Justice Statistics*. November 2014. Accessed August 19, 2017.

45 "Domestic Violence: Communities of Color." Oregon Department of Justice. June 2006. Accessed August 19, 2017.

46 Erika Harrell, PhD. "Black Victims of Violent Crime." *Bureau of Justice Statistics*. August 2007. Accessed August 19, 2017.

47 Perry, Steve W. "A BJS Statistical Profile, 1992-2002: American Indians and Crime." *Bureau of Justice Statistics*. December 2004. Accessed August 19, 2017.

48 David Cantor, Bonnie Fisher, Susan Chibnall, Reanna Townsend, et. al. "Report on the AAU Campus Climate Survey on Sexual Assault and Sexual Misconduct." *Westat*. September 2015. Accessed August 19, 2017.

education is the single biggest piece of the sexual assault issue that we need to change. To that end, they have the ROAR Back Program where, for each device sold, a portion of the proceeds goes toward educational programs that have been shown to increase empathy and reduce violence. Some of the organizations reaping the benefits of this program include Women Against Abuse, Women Organized Against Rape, Lutheran Settlement House, and One Love Foundation. "If we sell a lot and don't move the needle in regards [sic] to assault against women," says Gold, "we've failed."

For those who can't afford a device like the Athena, there are phone apps like Circle of 6, which operate in a similar way. A free app, users can tap icons to look up health and safety resources; send a text to their circle that says, "come and get me," containing their GPS location; send a text that says, "call and pretend you need me;" or send a text that says, simply, "I need to talk." The app uses icons so that it's not obvious to others that you're sending out a distress signal. You can also pre-program your app to call a hotline who can help in the case of rape or sexual assault.

The tech world is growing rich with resources such as these. Project Consent, for example, is an ongoing online campaign and community that uses social media to advocate for a future in which rape culture has been dismantled. They came onto my radar when I was managing social media for Good in Bed. Their sex ed graphics and videos were highly tweetable, and I dug how they were raising awareness around the shifting definition of consent in a way that was engaging and accessible.

For example, one video series featured animated, dancing genitalia, whose primary message was that, "Consent is simple. If it's not a yes, it's a no." Another series of graphics featured "#pawsoff," emblazoned across images of adorable dogs. More recently, they collaborated with apparel company Believe Me, which was started by two women who were sick of the normalization of sexual violence. Part of their proceeds go toward the New York City Alliance Against Sexual Assault.

Sarah Li started Project Consent in 2014. At the time, Project Consent was just an Instagram page where people could talk about their experiences and feelings around consent. Social media director Mackenzie Cakebread says it's only grown from there, with the impetus remaining for it to be a safe space for people to learn and discuss what's happening in their lives, and why issues of consent are so important.

Before becoming a staffer, Cakebread followed Project Consent's content online, regularly sharing their posts. "I thought the work they were doing was so amazing," she says. "Women the same age as me had gone through so much, but they were not going to let these experiences drag them down. Instead, they were uplifting themselves, and uplifting other people. I thought, 'Oh my god. I have to be a part of that.'"

Now, Project Consent is much more than its Instagram page. They're sharing content across a number of social networks including Twitter, Facebook, and Tumblr. On top of that, they've started developing sex ed curricula and other resources for those who want to make a difference in their own community. "Our main goal is 100 percent education," says Cakebread. "We all came from backgrounds where we were not taught sex ed in school. Or the sex ed was more fear-based. We're very much about educating people that you have a choice: you're allowed to say no; you're allowed to say yes; here's what you can do if you feel you can't say no. We want to make sure people know that there are options for them no matter what circumstances they're in."

Taking another approach is Capptivation, Inc., the company behind the Reach Out app. A free smart-phone app, it connects its users with resources such as rape crisis centers, helplines, legal aid services, medical care providers, counseling services, and emergency responders in their area.

The app's creators—a group of friends who had known each other since middle and high school—became curious about what they could do after reading the later retracted *Rolling Stone* article, "A Rape on Campus." Despite questions as to the veracity of the story,[49] the statistics it contained on campus assault were still eye-opening to them. "That was kind of preposterous to us," says Jack Zandi, one of Cappti-vation's founding partners. "I couldn't fathom one out of every five women[50] [on college campuses] being assaulted. That didn't seem possible because, if the stats were true . . . how is this not on every news channel

49 Sheila Coronel, Steve Coll, and Derek Kravitz. "Rolling Stone and UVA: The Columbia University Graduate School of Journalism Report." *Rolling Stone*, April 5, 2015.

50 Christopher P. Krebs PhD, Christine Lindquist, Marcus Berzovsky, Bonnie Shook-Sa, Kimberly Peterson, Michael Planty, Lynn Langton, and Jessica Stroop. "Campus Climate Survey Validation Study Final Technical Report." January 2016. Accessed August 21, 2017.

every day 24/7 until that number is zero? One in five means everyone knows someone. Literally."

So they created an app to help those who had been assaulted by enabling them to more easily find local and on-campus resources for talking to an advocate, getting medical attention, reporting the incident, and even for finding healing afterward. "The goal was to try to reduce the amount of inconveniences a survivor might come up against," says Zandi. "Anything could be enough to dissuade a survivor from reporting an assault. We're trying to give people more of a chance to get the help they need and maybe, as a result, the person who assaulted them will get caught."

By the time this book is published, I imagine there will be many more apps out there that enable women to take charge of their safety, their story, their healing. There will be more online communities. More educational campaigns. More tools. The number of tech tools being developed by and for women with the aim of protecting them or emboldening them or healing them is exploding. It is surreal to remember that none of this existed for us not that long ago.

Which is what flashed across my mind as I clipped my Athena to the neckline of my tank top at the end of yet another self-defense class, still not entirely used to its being there. After making sure it was secure, I hefted my bag over my shoulder, waved goodbye to my classmates, and walked downstairs, pushing open the gate where I had been buzzed in just two and a half hours earlier. It was dark, and I was in a neighborhood that was still unfamiliar to me, and I was alone. I was a little bit afraid, because I am always a little bit afraid when

I have to walk the streets on my own. But I had used my ROAR app before heading out, just so my contacts would be aware of where I was. And in my right hand, my keys poked out through my knuckles. My left hand was empty and twitching toward my safety device. My ears were still ringing with the *kiais* with which we had ended class, those guttural shouts we uttered with each practice strike. Whatever might happen, I was ready.

While I was a bundle of nerves the first time I drove into Brooklyn to learn blocks and kicks and palm strikes— *Will I find parking? Will I make it there on time? Will I be the most uncoordinated person there? Will I have to role play??*—I found myself looking forward to class in the succeeding weeks. And this despite the fact that I had to leave my home at 4:15 p.m. on a work day to get there by 6:30. As we lined up in two rows in the dojo, facing a mirrored wall, I gained confidence with every target they called out, my legs sure as they kicked the air in front of me, my arms strong as I threw them up to block my face. When we practiced wrist releases, my partner nodded approvingly as I whipped my arm around, sending them off balance. When we practiced the "butt up," the move I had performed so success-fully with my husband the week before, my partner flew backward, clutching her gut.

As galvanized as I felt every time we closed class with our concluding *kiais* and I descended to the street, the fact remained that the Center's very existence was a reaction to a culture we cannot seem to change. And as impressed as I was by ROAR for Good and the other tech companies that were carving out a space for women's safety and education and catharsis, this was also reactive.

In the past several years, I had become more interested and involved in sex ed advocacy. Part of this came from having worked for AASECT and learning through my work with them about the challenges educators face and the ways in which they meet these challenges. Part of this came from being the mother to a three-year-old girl. Teaching women to protect themselves from dangers that exist both within and outside the home was one thing. I wanted to create a world in which that danger no longer existed. Where I didn't have to be afraid for my daughter. Gold was right. Education was the biggest piece of the puzzle.

After talking with numerous sexuality educators, I'm convinced that comprehensive sexuality education is the key and that it needs to start earlier than high school. Only with this approach can the newer generations internalize the lessons about respect and boundaries and bodily autonomy they need before they become sexually active. But as of this writing, we live in a world in which our president has chosen to cut over $200 million in funding from teen pregnancy prevention programs,[51] which include sex education programs and classes that teach parents how to speak to their kids about sex. Instead, he is proposing that the government funnel $277 million toward abstinence-only

---

51 Jane Kay. "Trump administration suddenly pulls plug on teen pregnancy programs." Reveal. July 14, 2017. Accessed August 20, 2017. https://www.revealnews.org/article/trump-administration -suddenly-pulls-plug-on-teen-pregnancy-programs/.

education programs,[52] programs that have been shown to be ineffective.[53] Are we living in the darkest timeline? We certainly seem to be moving toward it.

While some educators feel strongly that consent education should only be one part of a larger educational foundation, the truth of the matter is that at this point it's often better than what many have received growing up. Is it any surprise that many of the educators developing consent education programs for students outside of traditional, school-based sex ed have themselves been touched by intimate partner violence or sexual assault or harassment?

I learned about YES! (Your Empowered Sexuality) when controversy erupted close to home over a planned abstinence-focused presentation at a local middle school. The story ended up in the local paper,[54] and YES! was presented as a welcome alternative to what was seen as a problematic program. The story mentioned that YES! was hosting a workshop for parents on how to discuss sex and puberty with teens and tweens. Though I'd already missed the workshop, I was excited to learn that such a group existed in my very own backyard, and

---

52 "Budget Of The U. S. Government A New Foundation for American Greatness: Fiscal Year 2018." The White House. Accessed August 20, 2017.

53 Kathrin F. Stanger-Hall and David W. Hall. "Abstinence-Only Education and Teen Pregnancy Rates: Why We Need Comprehensive Sex Education in the U.S." Edited by Virginia J. Vitzthum. *PLoS One* 6, no. 10 (October 14, 2011). doi:10.1371/journal.pone.0024658.

54 Erin Roll. "Sex education talk raises concerns among Glenfield parents." June 30, 2017. Accessed August 20, 2017. http://www.montclairlocal.news/wp/index.php/2017/05/04/montclair-sex-education-talk-raises-concerns-among-glenfield-parents/.

that it was created by a group of young women who clearly kicked ass. I immediately contacted them and ended up chatting with Isy Abraham-Raveson, one of the founding members and the group's dedicated curriculum writer.

Abraham-Raveson got her B.A. in Women's, Gender, and Sexuality studies, and wrote her thesis on sex education and sexual shame. Later, she was trained as a sexuality educator at the Masakhane Center in Newark, New Jersey, a sex ed organization only about twenty minutes away from where I live.

Abraham-Raveson tells me that she and a group of her high school friends—all recently graduated from college—returned home with the sense that they had gained a lot and now wanted to give back to their former high school and their community. They decided that consent workshops were something that aligned with their skill sets and that this type of education was something teens in their hometown weren't getting in school.

Though it was difficult getting administrators to allow them into the high schools, they eventually began working with after school clubs, such as the high school's Gay-Straight Alliance, in order to circumvent the usual bureaucracy. Eventually, as their reputation grew, the local public and private schools started inviting them in to teach workshops, and they began offering presentations to parents as well.

"It's devastating, the emotion of thinking you are inherently bad," says Abraham-Raveson, "and the fact that sexual shame is part of the norm for women—that it is not an unusual experience—is frightening. [The lack of education] is such a missed opportunity, because I think with good sex education and good communication and positivity, people can grow up feeling good about themselves."

Abraham-Raveson also believes that college-level consent education programs are just too little, too late. "Sexual assault happens in high school," she says. "The sooner you talk about it, the better. Students deserve to have that information. I didn't have sexual trauma, but I still felt so alienated from my body. It's so much easier to prevent all that from forming than to undo it later."

When I learned about YES!, they were only about a year old, and I ended up attending a silent auction they hosted at a favorite café of mine in order to raise money for the non-profit's expansion plans. They told attendees about their grand plans for additional chapters, curriculum development, and video production. They mentioned the community blog where people could share sex and body stories, whether painful or celebratory or healing. And they gave a shout-out to the coloring book they'd created—downloadable for free on their website—so that younger kids could learn about bodily autonomy.

"We're working toward a point where the school district knows we're a resource," says Abraham-Raveson, "and doesn't see us as an oppositional force. That's kinda the dream."

"So often, adults think adolescent sexuality is something to be controlled," she continues. "They want to protect these girls. But what are their experiences? What questions do they have? We're creating a space for people to talk about it openly. I just think that this model of reclaiming sexuality is what most of us went through and, best case scenario, we're hoping they never have that moment where they have to reclaim it, because they never lost it."

But with one in every six women having experienced sexual assault,[55] that path toward reclamation is still relevant and necessary. The Australia-based South Eastern Centre Against Sexual Assault & Family Violence lists powerlessness, loss of control, and loss of sexual confidence[56] as just some of the reactions to sexual assault. And while there is research showing that hypersexuality is a common reaction to sexual trauma,[57] the opposite (which I experienced) is also true. Those who have been assaulted often avoid sex afterward as their satisfaction and pleasure in sexual activities diminishes.[58] And one study shows that fear responses—including dissociation—can replay over and over again for sexual assault victims every time they feel triggered.[59] Which is why programs that enable victims to cross that chasm of

55 "Victims of Sexual Violence: Statistics." RAINN. Accessed August 14, 2017. https://www.rainn.org/statistics/victims-sexual-violence.

56 "Feelings after sexual assault." Accessed August 30, 2017. https://www.secasa.com.au/pages/feelings-after-sexual-assault/.

57 Mark F. Schwartz, ScD, Lori D. Galperin, LCSW, and William H. Masters, MD. "Post-Traumatic Stress, Sexual Trauma and Dissociative Disorder." National Institute of Justice. March 17, 1995.

58 Willy Van Berlo and Bernardine Ensink. "Problems with Sexuality after Sexual Assault." *Annual Review of Sex Research* 11, no. 1 (2000): 235-67.

59 Maggie Schauer and Thomas Elbert. "Dissociation Following Traumatic Stress." *Zeitschrift für Psychologie / Journal of Psychology* 218, no. 2 (2010): 109-27. doi:10.1027/0044-3409/a000018.

disconnect between themselves and their bodies are so important.

Empowerment self-defense courses go a long way toward accomplishing this. But as restorative as they were for me, self-defense classes are primarily intended to prevent future assault. And as I conducted research for this book, I became curious about what existed that was specifically intended to help survivors *heal*.

I found some interesting approaches.

For example, there are a slew of tattoo artists who dedicate a portion of their work hours to inking over people's domestic violence scars, and others who simply provide tattoos to those who have experienced sexual violence as a way of allowing them to regain control of their bodies, providing them with a permanent reminder that they are no longer victims, but are survivors.[60] Which is cool, considering how research shows that body art can have a positive emotional, physical, and sexual effect on those who have experienced abuse.[61]

As a yoga practitioner and teacher who came to the practice at a difficult time and found it to be a life raft, I was especially interested in trauma-informed yoga classes. Which is why, one Monday evening, I drove into Bushwick for one of the few classes I found that

---

60 Patty Branco. "Reclaiming the body after trauma: Can body art help abuse survivors heal?" VAWnet. April 3, 2017. http://vawnet. org/news/reclaiming-body-after-trauma-can-body-art-help-abuse-survivors-heal.

61 Jerome R. Koch, Alden E. Roberts, Myrna L. Armstrong, and Donna C. Owen. "Tattoos, gender, and well-being among American college students." *The Social Science Journal* 52, no. 4 (August 28, 2015): 536–41. doi:10.1016/j.soscij.2015.08.001.

was open to the public. The event was offered by the folks behind Exhale to Inhale, an organization that uses volunteer instructors to bring yoga to survivors of domestic violence and sexual assault through their free classes at shelters and other locations. That evening, we gathered in a narrow gallery space, our mats lined up along one wall. Latin music drifted in through the open doorway and the sound of the subway roared overhead every few minutes.

As we moved through the practice, I found it not too different from the yoga I tried to teach my own students, the yoga I practiced on my own mat. Yes, the language was more invitational than the language that was used at my home studio, and we were encouraged to play with movement in order to find what worked for us. Yes, the instructor eschewed hands-on adjustments in favor of allowing us to follow what our bodies were calling out for. But for the most part, I was able to sink easily into what was familiar. Which is why I find yoga to be such a grounding practice.

But what is it that makes a yoga class trauma-informed, and what might my fellow practitioners have been experiencing during that hour of movement and breath?

According to David Emerson, the founder and director of Yoga Services at the Trauma Center at the Justice Resource Institute in Brookline, Massachusetts, trauma-informed yoga is primarily about power, and about how we deal with varying power dynamics. For example, there is the language instructors use. "Instead of telling people what to do," says Emerson, "we say, 'if you like' or, 'maybe put your left foot forward, possibly raising your arms.' The whole teacher-student relation-ship is built around that invitational approach."

Another important aspect of classes is the lack of importance placed upon the poses—or "forms"—and upon how we think they're "supposed to" look. "They don't matter so much," says Emerson. "There is no specific form we do for any particular purpose. They all provide equal opportunities to do a couple things: to practice invitational relationships, and to practice choice making." To that end, instructors are trained to be clear about the various options students have when practicing a form, as those who have experienced trauma, and who are experiencing PTSD as a result, often have impaired body awareness.[62] "We know people have a hard time taking in information and figuring out what to do. How to actualize that in their own bodies," says Emerson.

In speaking about the benefits the practice can have, Emerson mentions how the practice is intended to give people agency, allowing them to do things for themselves in safe way, a freedom that is lost in a coercive, manipu-lative, or otherwise abusive relationship. "We want to use these forms as chances to interact, to access those wants for real," says Emerson. "Someone can acknowl-edge to themselves, 'It's uncomfortable for me to twist this much, so I can twist less.' This reclamation of agency is a very important part of the healing process."

The practice also strengthens interoception, which is

---

62 Jennifer West, Belle Liang, and Joseph Spinazzola. "Trauma sensitive yoga as a complementary treatment for posttraumatic stress disorder: A qualitative descriptive analysis." *International Journal of Stress Management* 24, no. 2 (July 4, 2016): 173–95. doi:10.1037/str0000040.

the ability to feel or sense what the body is experiencing. "Hunger is an example," says Emerson. "Feeling our heart beat. The parts of the brain that transfer these pieces of information from the body to awareness are— for traumatized people—very dysregulated. Because it hasn't been safe to feel the body. To experience too much when being abused or neglected. This yoga practice gives students the opportunity to have these visceral experiences in a contained way. To practice noticing what they feel and telling themselves, 'As long as I can tolerate that, I'll do it. If not, I can stop.'"

Emerson cites the research of psychiatrist Judith Lewis Herman, who wrote in her book *Trauma and Recovery*,[63] "No intervention that takes power away from the survivor can possibly foster her recovery."

"If we're not dealing with power first," says Emerson, "we're not gonna get anywhere. We're not gonna help anyone."

In research conducted through the Trauma Center on finding peaceful embodiment through yoga in the aftermath of trauma,[64] participants reported feelings of safety, calm, groundedness, presence, inner strength, and self-confidence. The paper—eventually published in *Complementary Therapies in Clinical Practice*— is filled with powerful participant testimonials. One participant reported:

---

63 Judith Lewis Herman. *Trauma and recovery: aftermath of violence from domestic abuse to political terror.* New York: BasicBooks, 2015.

64 Alison M. Rhodes. "Claiming peaceful embodiment through yoga in the aftermath of trauma." *Complementary Therapies in Clinical Practice* 21, no. 4 (2015): 247-56. doi:10.1016/j.ctcp.2015.09.004.

When you are abused you feel small, even smaller than you are. That was my experience as a child. I wanted to be small and invisible if possible. I wanted not to be seen, and I constricted . . . I'd say the sense of being able to open up in this way physically [in yoga], as simple as it sounds, especially the upper part of my body—heart, lungs, diaphragm, shoulders—all the parts that I had scrunched down, that seemed to make a difference. It allowed an overall expansion.

Another participant reported on the positive effects the practice had on her relationship to others:

The most important thing was being able to connect, and not being fearful to connect because there were times when I couldn't. One example is that [the yoga teacher] got me to stretch my arms out even with my shoulders, which I had not been able to do. It was a fear. And the thing that I notice the most is because I was able to extend my arms out I was able to hug people, to invite someone to have a hug. [This made me feel] happy. Because it's bodywork, I could learn to accept being touched by others in a different way, and that has enhanced some relationships, especially the one with my husband. Because sexual intimacy has been messed up for me . . . I was a mess, but now I can actually be intimate with someone I want to be intimate with. Even if it's just cuddly, and I don't need to be afraid of his touch or threatened by it, and actually enjoy it, not numb out or shut down.

"It's about giving yourself permission," said our instructor that evening in Brooklyn, referring to the permission to move or not move in a certain way. To feel or not feel.

I feel lucky to have found yoga when I did. To have developed a body awareness that allows me to know when something is wrong. To know when my body is thirsting for one thing instead of another. Seven years in, I have no problem giving myself permission to do a supported bridge or shoulder stand, or to recline in legs up the wall, or to take a modification of a pose that seems as if it will be better for my body. The classes I took—and am still taking—were not strictly trauma-informed but, by that point, I had spent years reacting to my own experience through other means: through sexual exploration, and small feats of courage, and through the shock therapy that my sex writing became for me.

For those who don't have this, a practice like trauma-informed yoga seems a far less circuitous route to healing and reclamation.

Meanwhile, I found that through all of my research, the intervention I connected to the most was empowerment self-defense, probably thanks to that strong foundation of body awareness I already gained through yoga. I found myself bereft as my last class drew to a close, unsure that I would be capable of carrying all of its lessons with me into the future.

One of the exercises we conducted during that last class required that we walk through a gauntlet of our classmates, using the techniques we learned in the previous weeks to fend off multiple assailants. As I stood at the head of those two parallel lines of people, I was asked to close my eyes so that my instructor could tap a handful of my classmates, marking them as my attackers. I vibrated with anxiety. Practicing a specific move with a partner was one thing. Being unaware of where an attack would be coming from, and what form it would take, was another thing entirely.

I was tense when I opened my eyes and crept forward. The first attacker came from behind and grabbed me around my middle. I dragged him around the room, trying to do the "butt up" over and over again, unable to get enough leverage to simultaneously lift my arms and push him away. In hindsight, I should have elbowed him in the solar plexus but, instead, I eventually used my voice, and he melted back into line.

I was still shaken when the next attacker came up behind me and drew an arm around my neck. But I was able to elbow her in the gut, spin around, and thrust the heel of my hand toward her nose, warding her off.

The final attacker also grabbed me from behind. This time, when I did the "butt up," she flew backwards, ending my trial. I trembled with relief. I had made it through the gauntlet. While I hadn't performed perfectly, I'd at least done it. My upper arms throbbed from where my first attacker had held me tight, and I knew bruises would surface there later on. The ache reminded me that there was still work to be done. I had to continue practicing, internalizing the lessons I'd learned until I was able to move with pure instinct.

Our final act of that evening—and the culmination of our five weeks together—was board breaking. All of the anxiety I experienced before my very first class came rushing back. *What if I embarrass myself? What if I hurt myself? What if I'm the only person who fails to break their board and everyone points at me and says neener-neener?*

I'm ashamed to say that as I watched classmate after classmate walk to the front of the room and place their board on top of two bricks, I hoped that someone would fail. Anyone. Just so I wouldn't be the only one.

As each person made their way up there—as each person broke their board—I curled deeper into myself, queasy and clammy and afraid to raise my hand to go next.

But finally, I was the only one left. So I pushed myself to my feet, slunk up to the front of the room, and took the board my instructor handed to me. I chose a purple marker and drew a smiling cat at the center of my board to give myself a point of focus. I placed my board atop the two bricks and stepped back, placing my feet hip-width apart, lifting my arms. *One* – I inhaled in and out through my nose, placed the edge of my hand on that cat's face, let my vision shrink down to a pinpoint – *two* – I inhaled to draw my hand back again, exhaled as I placed it back down – *three!* – "KIAI!" I shouted, and my hand flew down, and the board flew apart, breaking right down the center.

My legs were wobbly as I walked back to my spot, clutching my two pieces of board to my body, the rest of my classmates applauding. I sat down and placed the pieces on the ground in front of me, stared at them as our instructors brought the class to a close.

Shock. Strength. Pride. These were all things I felt as I rubbed a finger across the board's surface.

Shock. Strength. Pride. These are all things I feel as I move forward.

But mixed in with those emotions are other feelings, too. More complicated feelings. Frustration that, despite change, it is still not enough. Enduring fear, for both myself and my daughter. Anger. So much anger.

But then there is also hope.

"What's the title of your book?" my mom asked me the other day, during a phone call.

"*A Dirty Word,*" I told her, trying to ignore the fact that my book deal had been announced four months ago, for the love of god.

"No it is not!" she said, implying that I was joking.

"Yes, it is," I insisted, trying to explain the multiple meanings in the title, the ways in which we often demonize female sexuality.

She lowered her voice, as if we were exchanging deep and dirty secrets. "Is this a book your daughter is going to be embarrassed by?" she asked me next.

"I hope not!"

I didn't say aloud that her question was the reason I had to write it.

As things stand now, I think Michael and I are doing a pretty good job of ensuring she won't be embarrassed.

"Do I have a penis?" Emily asked me just the other month.

I stifled a laugh. "Nope," I said. "You don't have a penis. You have a vagina and a vulva! Girls have vaginas and vulvas. Boys have penises." I was repeating lessons she'd already learned from *Who Has What?*, a Robie H. Harris book we sometimes read together before bed.

"You have a vagina?" persisted Emily.

"Yup! I have a vagina."

"And I have a vagina," she confirmed.

"Yup."

She paused to take all of this this in. And then: "Do you have a butt?"

"I sure do," I said.

"And I have a butt, too," she said, clearly elated. "We all have butts!"

Butts for everyone! I thought.

Even though I have spoken with scores of brilliant sex educators, even though I have taught teens how to use writing as advocacy, even though I have reconnected with my body through yoga, even though I have learned empowerment self-defense and broken my board . . . it is her.

She is the one who gives me hope. She is the reason I still write. She is the proof that things can be different.

For her, sex will never be a dirty word.

Or at least that is the thing I strive for.

APPENDIX

If it isn't already obvious, I'm the type of person who believes in self-education as a means of improving one's life. When I was struggling with a shopping problem, and the attendant credit card debt, I picked up books on personal finance. Before I ditched my job in book publishing to go full-time freelance, I read a shit-ton of books on freelance writing, business-building, and entrepreneurship. I attacked my sex life in much the same way. This book is a record of that.

Because I don't want to leave you with anecdote alone—as helpful and reassuring as that can be—here's a list of resources you can use if you're trying to find fulfillment or reclamation in your own sex life. Feel free to mark up and dog-ear these pages. That's what I would do.

AMAZE, amaze.org. A sex ed video series everyone and their mother has been raving about, this initiative is a collaboration between groups such as Advocates for Youth, the Center for Reproductive Rights, Planned Parenthood, Rise Up, SIECUS, Scarleteen, and other awesome organizations I'd like to give all my money to.

American Association of Sexuality Educators Counselors and Therapists (AASECT), aasect.org. A professional organization for sexuality professionals, you can use AASECT's online member directory to locate a clinician near you.

Babeland, babeland.com. Babeland, my favorite female-friendly sex shop, has locations in Seattle, Brooklyn, and Manhattan. Like any other cute boutique you might enter, the décor is bright and fun, and the staff is friendly and knowledgeable. They also have sample units of their toys on display so you can test the intensity of vibration, feel the heft of a toy in your hand, and basically make the best possible purchasing decision for you. All locations also offer a variety of continuing sexuality education events. If you don't live nearby, don't worry. You can purchase all of their products online.

Bad Feminist, **by Roxane Gay.** Gay's collection is about many things, including race and pop culture and even competitive scrabble. But there is also much to read here about gender and femininity, safety and sexual violence. Gay is brilliant about all of it, bringing her sharp eye, quiet humor, and a sense of solid matter-of-factness to everything she explores.

Because It Feels Good: A Woman's Guide to Sexual Pleasure and Satisfaction, **by Debby Herbenick, PhD.** Herbenick—a research scientist at Indiana University, a sexual health educator at the Kinsey Institute, and a widely read sex columnist—manages mysexprofessor.com, a media company sharing information on sex, sexual health, and relationships. But it was her book—a "pleasure manifesto" and guide to a great sex life—that made me a fan for life.

Betty Dodson with Carlin Ross, dodsonandross.com. Betty Dodson is an artist and author with a PhD in sexology and a private sex coaching practice. Carlin Ross is a sex educator. Together, they run a sex-positive, feminist website rife with how-to videos, podcasts, and more.

Center for Anti-Violence Education, caeny.org. An organization that develops and implements violence prevention programs, this is where I took my own five-week empowerment self-defense class. In addition to the adult self-defense class I took (offered to victims of domestic violence and sexual assault for free), they also teach an after-school program for teen women and trans youth, karate, tai chi, and more. I'd keep going there myself forever and ever if the drive into Brooklyn wasn't such a bitch.

Center for Sexual Health Promotion, sexualhealth. indiana.edu. The center is a collaborative of sexual health scholars from across the campuses of Indiana University and other academic institutions. Participants work toward advancing the field of sexual health through research, education, and training initiatives.

Cinderella Ate My Daughter: Dispatches from the Front Lines of the New Girlie-Girl Culture, **by Peggy Orenstein.** What Orenstein refers to as girlie-girl culture is really just a capitalistic attempt to cash in on culturally-based gender norms. This is a fascinating read, especially if you're a new parent still trying to figure out what to teach your own daughter. Orenstein's follow-up, *Girls & Sex: Navigating the Complicated New Landscape,* is also killer.

Circle of 6, circleof6app.com. This is a free phone app that allows you to discreetly alert your emergency contacts if you feel you're in danger.

***Come as You Are: The Surprising New Science That Will Transform Your Sex Life,* by Emily Nagoski, PhD.** A book that focuses on the latest research on female sexual desire and makes it accessible to the lay person, *Come as You Are* is what led me to the epiphany that I am normal. That I am not dysfunctional. That I am not broken. That I can have as much (or as little) sex as I damn well please.

Defend Yourself, defendyourself.org. For another source of empowerment self-defense, this D.C.-based organization offers classes on self-defense and bystander intervention.

Exhale to Inhale, exhaletoinhale.org. This organization offers yoga classes at domestic violence shelters and community centers throughout New York City, the Hudson Valley, Connecticut, and Los Angeles. These classes are intended to empower women who have experienced intimate partner violence and sexual assault to heal and reclaim their lives.

***For Goodness Sex,* by Al Vernacchio.** This is the book other sexuality educators rave about, and when I saw Vernacchio give a presentation at the National Sex Ed

Conference, I finally understood why: he is brilliant and funny and his methods for teaching adolescents about puberty are amazing. This book lays out his approach to sex ed and offers adults the tools they need to approach the topic with their kids.

From Diapers to Dating: A Parent's Guide to Raising Sexually Healthy Children, **by Debra Haffner.** Laid out in sections organized by age group, Haffner's book gives parents a solid plan for what they should be teaching their children as they make their way through baby-hood, toddlerhood and, eventually, tweenhood. It also includes a kick-ass appendix (clearly, I *love* appendices) for books your children can read as the years go by.

Good in Bed, goodinbed.com. Full disclosure: Good in Bed is a client of mine. *52 Weeks of Amazing Sex* was the first project I did for them, and I've ghostwritten and edited a handful of other books on the site. In addition to e-books, the site offers expert advice on sexuality, active forums, scientific sexual research, and other resources. Good in Bed was founded by sex counselor Ian Kerner, PhD, a sex and relationships counselor and the best-selling author of *She Comes First*.

Guttmacher Institute, guttmacher.org. As a journalist in the areas of women's health and sexuality, I need to stay on top of the latest research on trends in reproductive health. The Guttmacher Institute tends to be one of my primary sources of statistics on abortion, contraception, education, and more.

Hunger, **by Roxane Gay.** A book about Gay's relationship with her body, this work of prose poetry blew me away. In it, Gay opens herself up in a way she never has before, splaying herself across the page as she tackles issues of the body, sexual violence, and self-worth.

Jimmyjane's Iconic Smoothie, jimmyjane.com/shop/iconicsmoothie-p-118.html. Though my first love was the Water Dancer, Jimmyjane's Iconic Smoothie is my new go-to vibrator. Simple in design, this battery-powered, waterproof, plastic vibe can be used for both clitoral and vaginal stimulation.

Juicebox, juiceboxit.com. There have been a slew of smartphone apps launching lately as alternatives to traditional, school-based sexuality education. One of the ones that has really caught my eye is Juicebox, which allows teens to ask sexual health experts their questions, anonymously. It seems like a great resource for those who are nervous about asking their teachers, their health care providers, or even their parents about the things they're most curious about.

Kate McCombs, M.P.H., katemccombs.com. I first fell in platonic love with sexuality educator Kate McCombs—and her teaching style—after seeing her in a video about creating what she refers to as "beacon of permission" moments: moments in which it feels safe to have a meaningful conversation about sex. I'm still waiting for her to write a book but, until then, you can read her blog or attend one of her sexuality workshops.

The Kinsey Institute for Research in Sex, Gender, and Reproduction, kinseyinstitute.org. Infamous for the Kinsey Report (*Kinsey's Sexual Behavior in the Human Male*), the development of which was dramatized in the 2004 biopic starring Liam Neeson (and the absolutely yummy Peter Sarsgaard), the Kinsey Institute is still doing amazing work, advancing sexual health and knowledge around the world. The Institute does this through a number of programs, including an active research program, library and art collections, research publications, and events, and also a sexuality information service called Kinsey Confidential (kinseyconfidential.org).

Lighter Than My Shadow, **by Katie Green.** I picked up a copy of this graphic memoir at Book Expo America (BEA), and it was the heaviest book in my tote bag. Lugging it around the city and all the way back home turned out to be worth it, though. About sexual abuse and eating disorders and depression, Green's work had me silently weeping.

Logan Levkoff, PhD, loganlevkoff.com. I was first introduced to Logan by a fellow sex writer when I was in my mid-twenties. She is an AASECT-certified sex educator with a PhD in Human Sexuality, Marriage, and Family Life Education from New York University, as well as an MS in Human Sexuality Education from the University of Pennsylvania. She works with students of all ages and from a variety of backgrounds, providing sexuality education in many independent schools and community organizations. A recognized expert on sexuality and relationships, Levkoff encourages honest conversation about sexuality. In other words, she's a woman after my own heart. When she asked me to edit her Good in Bed eBook, *How to Get Your Wife to Have Sex with You*, in 2011, I almost died of fangirl-ness. I look forward to eventually referencing her latest book, *Got Teens? The Doctor Mom's Guide to Sexuality, Social Media and Other Adolescent Realities*.

Mean, by Myriam Gurba. I read this book for a two-person book club that is just me and one of my besties. A lyrical, coming-of-age memoir, the beauty of Gurba's words contrasted sharply with the ugliness of her experiences, and with her brazen honesty around her interior world. Among other things, the book tackles sexual violence, guilt, culpability, race, misogyny, and homophobia.

Men Explain Things to Me, by Rebecca Solnit. This book is a call to action for those embroiled in the worldwide war on women. In the broadest sense, Solnit's book is about the gender wars, but the two pieces that really donkey-kicked me in the gut were the ones that tackled domestic violence and sexual assault. Reading this slim collection was like hearing a rallying cry. It should be required reading for all men and women.

Moregasm: Babeland's Guide to Mind-Blowing Sex, by Rachel Venning, Claire Cavanah, and Jessica Vitkus. Authored by the peeps behind my favorite sex shop, *Moregasm* is the type of book that should appear on sexuality education curricula everywhere and be passed out during college orientations. A manual of modern sex, it's filled with stylish photographs and illustrations, questions, suggestions, personal stories from real people, and easy-to-follow advice.

My Body Back Project, mybodybackproject.com. I am *so all about* this London-based group that works with women who have experienced sexual violence, helping them to reconnect with their bodies. They offer cervical screening, maternity care, discussion groups, and more. I have yet to find one quite like it here in the U.S., but I'm sure it's out there. And if you know about it, I want you to let *me* know so I can share it with the world!

Our Bodies, Ourselves, **by the Boston Women's Health Book Collective and Judy Norsigian.** Another must for any sexuality education curriculum, *Our Bodies, Ourselves* is a sexual health classic. Its contents give women everything they need for making key decisions about their health, from definitive information from today's leading experts to personal stories from other women just like them. This means comprehensive information on relationships, sexuality, and sexual health; reproductive choices, pregnancy, and childbearing; and more. Together with its companion website (www.ourbodiesourselves.org), *Our Bodies, Ourselves* is a one-stop resource for women of all generations.

Planned Parenthood, plannedparenthood.org. Full disclosure: I blog on a freelance basis for my local Planned Parenthood affiliate, the Center for Sex Education. That's because I believe PP is an indispensable resource for sexuality education, sexual health services, contraceptive access, and affordable health care.

Project Consent, projectconsent.com. The people behind the dancing genital videos, PC is an online campaign and community who use social media in order to advocate for a future in which rape culture has been dismantled. Follow them on Twitter, Tumblr, Instagram . . . they're all over the damn place, creating consent-focused campaigns that make people sit up and take notice.

Reach Out app, capptivation.com. This free app—created mostly for college students—gives its users access to local resources they can use if they have been sexually assaulted.

ROAR for Good, roarforgood.com. The developers of the Athena device and the app it pairs with, this organization also raises money for sex ed programs whose purpose is to get to the root of rape culture. Purchase a piece of safety jewelry at their website in order to both support their cause and also feel an eensy bit safer.

Scarleteen, scarleteen.com. This is the sexuality education site I wish I knew about growing up. Scarleteen is an independent, grassroots sexuality education site for young women. It contains how-to content, message boards, mentoring, referrals for sexual/reproductive healthcare services, and more.

Seal Press, sealpress.com. Inspired by the simple yet radical notion that a book can change a woman's life,

Seal Press is devoted to publishing titles that inform, reveal, engage, delight, and support women of all ages and backgrounds. Their backlist includes titles like *Healing Painful Sex, Good Porn, What You Really Really Want, Open, Getting Off, Naked on the Internet,* and basically everything else on my bookshelf.

Sex & Sensibility: The Thinking Parent's Guide to Talking Sense About Sex, by Deborah M. Roffman. I'm a huge fan of Roffman's friendly, open, and easygoing tone, bolstered by her own stories of missteps in the parenting trenches. Beyond this, she does a brilliant job of showing readers how to approach difficult topics with their children no matter their cultural or religious background, or their belief system.

Sex Is a Funny Word, by Cory Silverberg. For the younger set, this comic book for kids contains lessons about bodies, gender, and sexuality.

Sexuality Information and Education Council of the United States (SIECUS), siecus.org. SIECUS is an advocacy organization that provides education and information about sexuality and sexual and reproductive health.

Speak, by Laurie Halse Anderson. This book is a YA novel about a year in the life of a teenage girl who is sinking under the weight of a big, terrible secret: her rape at the hands of a high school senior the summer before. This book was gripping and true and heartbreaking and insightful and an important read for teen girls everywhere.

Trauma Center Trauma-Sensitive Yoga, traumasensi-tiveyoga.com. This center, located in Brookline, Massachusetts, is the birthplace of research-based, trauma-focused yoga instruction. What this means is that teachers who train here learn how to take an approach to the teaching of yoga that allows those who have suffered from trauma reclaim their bodies for themselves.

Who Has What? **by Robie H. Harris.** And basically everything else Harris has ever written. Sexuality educators swear by these children's books, and this particular one is in regular rotation during my daughter's bedtime. Leading to conversations between my daughter and my husband such as this one: Emily (after barging in on my husband peeing): Is that your penis? Michael: Yes, it's my penis. Emily: I don't have a penis. Michael: That's right. You have a vagina and a vulva. Emily: Mommy has a vagina and a vulva, too. Michael: [pees] Emily (who has yet to potty train): Good job!

Womankind, iamwomankind.org. I can't remember when I first learned about this group, but one of its staffers was at the trauma-informed yoga class I took in Brooklyn. They are an advocacy group who work with survivors of gender-based violence in order to lead them toward healing.

YES! (Your Empowered Sexuality), yestoconsent.org. This small, consent education organization formed by a group of young, kick-ass ladies brings consent education to teens and also provides opportunities for parents to learn how to approach sex-related conversations with their kids.

You Don't Have to Like Me: Essays on Growing Up, Speaking Out, and Finding Feminism, by Alida Nugent. This book is part of a crop of fierce, feminist manifestas that came out between 2014 and 2016. If nothing else, it is an accessible read for those who have yet to claim feminism for themselves.

ACKNOWLEDGMENTS

Fifteen years ago, I started writing about sex, and my parents weren't weird about it. Sure, my mom made it clear that she hoped this was all just a phase and that, someday, I'd write about something much more respectable. And my dad made dildo jokes. But my mom still made photocopies of my first print magazine clip (in *Playgirl*!) and passed them around to friends and coworkers, and my dad—well, he still made dildo jokes. So more than anyone else, I have to thank my parents for always being supportive of this thing I do, even though they don't always understand it.

And while we're at it, let me thank my brother, too. I can't imagine any of my family members actually wanting to *read* all of this but, by god, I know they'll all continue to support me no matter what.

I'd also like to thank my husband, Michael, for playing the guinea pig throughout the course of my sex writing career, and for allowing me to reveal so many intimate details about our life together through my writing.

Next up, I want to thank my daughter, Emily, who is still just a toddler. I want to thank her because—at a time when I was feeling burnt out on writing about sex, unsure of what the point of it all was—she gave me a renewed sense of purpose. If you've read this entire book, you know that I started out writing about sex in order to fix myself. I continue to write about sex in order to fix the world, primarily for my daughter's sake.

And then there's Lyz Lenz, my tireless writing partner, upon whom I am completely dependent. We've been working together for over seven years now, and I can't make a single, goddamn decision without her. Seriously. It's ridiculous. I wish she would relocate to New Jersey so I could visit her without warning with all of my writing conundrums. Though, actually, this would probably be a nightmare for Lyz.

I also need to thank my writing critique group, whom I connected with through the Montclair Write Group. We meet every Wednesday to swap feedback and, no joke, it is the highlight of my week. Much love to Melissa, Ren, Kyrce, Joanne, Debby, and Rose.

Of course, you wouldn't be reading any of this if it weren't for my agent, Sharon Pelletier of Dystel, Goderich & Bourret LLC, my editor, Hannah Bennett, my publicist, Allyson Fields, and the rest of the awesome team at Cleis Press and Start Publishing.

And just to be thorough, I want to thank all of my friends who continue to be my friends even though I write about the sexy sex, like, A LOT. Plus: all of the sexuality professionals who have inspired my work, most notably Emily Nagoski, whose brilliant and eye-opening *Come as You Are* changed the entire course of this book. And also my cats Gizmo, Kooshie, and Lusa, for only sitting on my keyboard 10 percent of the time.

Hugs! – Steph